WO 18·2 MCQ

300 Essential SBAs
in Surgery
with explanatory answers

KAJI SRITHARAN
Specialist Registrar in General Surgery
North West Thames, London Deanery

SAMIA IJAZ
Specialist Registrar in General Surgery
North West Thames, London Deanery

and

NEIL RUSSELL
Specialist Registrar in General Surgery
Eastern Deanery

Foreword by

TIM ALLEN-MERSH
Professor of Gastrointestinal Surgery
Chair, London NW Specialist Training Committee in General Surgery
Imperial College School of Medicine
Chelsea and Westminster Hospital, London

Radcliffe Publishing
Oxford • New York

Radcliffe Publishing Ltd
18 Marcham Road
Abingdon
Oxon OX14 1AA
United Kingdom

www.radcliffe-oxford.com
Electronic catalogue and worldwide online ordering facility.

British Library Cataloguing in Publication Data

A catalogue record for this book is available from the British Library.

ISBN-13: 978 1 84619 290 6

The paper used for the text pages of this book is FSC certified. FSC (The Forest Stewardship Council) is an international network to promote responsible management of the world's forests.

Mixed Sources
Product group from well-managed
forests and other controlled sources
www.fsc.org Cert no. SGS-COC-2482
© 1996 Forest Stewardship Council

Typeset by Pindar New Zealand, Auckland, New Zealand
Printed and bound by TJI Digital, Padstow, Cornwall, UK

Contents

Foreword

Examinations in medicine frequently include a multiple choice question (MCQ) component, because this form of assessment is regarded as fair, robust and defensible. I'm delighted that three outstanding surgical trainees have collaborated to produce *300 Essential SBAs in Surgery*. They are well placed to write these questions because they have recent experience of sitting MCQ papers and also of preparing medical students for final MB examinations in surgery.

The questions have been designed to cover the final MB surgical syllabus. As a result, they are clinically relevant and relate to topics – both clinical vignettes and knowledge-based scenarios – that frequently come up in these examinations. Some more difficult questions have been included, in order to challenge the more able student and to be relevant for MRCS Part A revision.

The answers have been provided in some detail, in order to leave the learner with an understanding of the background to the question. Opinion and evidence in medicine is always evolving, and MCQ question banks need to be kept up to date. The questions in *300 Essential SBAs in Surgery* are all new and relate to currently accepted standards of care in surgery.

I hope that *300 Essential SBAs in Surgery* will help you to get through your surgery exams and maybe even inspire you to a career in surgery!

Tim Allen-Mersh
Professor of Gastrointestinal Surgery
Chair, London NW Specialist Training Committee in General Surgery
Imperial College School of Medicine
Chelsea and Westminster Hospital, London
June 2009

Preface

The face of medical education and the tools by which it is assessed are continually evolving. Single best answer (SBA) questions are a relatively new method of assessment and are commonly encountered in the final MBBS surgical examination.

The key to success in any SBA-style examination is practice, practice and more practice, and this book is intended to provide just that. With 300 structured questions, it comprehensively covers the surgical curriculum. Each specialty-specific chapter contains a combination of clinical vignettes and knowledge-based questions of varying degrees of difficulty in order to both challenge the more able candidate and provide a realistic appreciation of the standard required to pass. Importantly, each question gives an explanation of the correct answer, and it is hoped that this will allow readers to reflect upon their choice of answer and reinforce their understanding of the topic.

This book is the ideal revision aid for all medical students studying towards their final MBBS examination in surgery. Doctors studying for the MRCS and PLAB examinations will also find this book extremely useful.

Kaji Sritharan
Samia Ijaz
Neil Russell
June 2009

About the authors

Kaji Sritharan studied medicine at St Mary's Hospital Medical School and was awarded an intercalated BSc in Physiology from University College London. She completed her basic surgical training in London and subsequently undertook an MD with the Department of Vascular Surgery, Charing Cross Hospital, and the Kennedy Institute of Rheumatology, Imperial College London. She is currently a specialist registrar in General Surgery on the North West Thames rotation.

Kaji has considerable teaching experience. She is currently president of the Trainees' Committee of the Royal Society of Medicine and has held posts as an anatomy demonstrator and as a tutor in anatomy and embryology at Christ Church College, University of Oxford. During her time in Oxford, she was involved in developing the Computer Assisted Learning Modules in Anatomy and Embryology and was awarded the Dooley Prize in Anatomy for her contribution to teaching. Kaji has also been a PBL tutor at Imperial College London; and here she was involved in both facilitating and organising the third-year Clinical OSCE and final MBBS Clinical Examinations in Surgery.

In addition, she has written extensively and is author of *Essential OSCE Topics for Medical and Surgical Finals* (Radcliffe Publishing, 2007), *Get Through Postgraduate Medical Interviews* (RSM Press, 2008), *Essential Notes for Medical and Surgical Finals* (Radcliffe Publishing, 2008) and Netter's online *Anatomy Lab*.

Samia Ijaz studied medicine at St Mary's Hospital Medical School, where she intercalated a BSc in Infection and Immunity. She completed her basic surgical training rotation in London and then undertook an MS research project for two years prior to starting higher surgical training on the North West Thames rotation in 2003.

Samia has been involved in teaching throughout her medical career to date. Specifically, following her pre-registration year she spent six months teaching anatomy to medical and dental students, anaesthetists and orthotists at Manchester University Medical School. She has also taught on several basic surgical skills courses and regularly takes final-year medical students through mock clinical OSCE stations.

Samia has been awarded her MS and has published numerous peer-reviewed articles in medical journals, based on her thesis and various clinical topics.

Neil Russell qualified as a doctor in 2001, having gained a BSc (Hons) in Medical Science from St Andrews University, before studying clinical medicine at Cambridge University, where he was a member of Emmanuel College. He spent his pre-registration house officer year in Cambridge and then went on to complete his basic surgical training in Nottingham. In March 2005 Neil gained his MRCS, and in August 2005 he returned to Cambridge to take up the position of clinical research fellow in Transplantation, working jointly with the Department of Surgery at Addenbrooke's Hospital and the Centre for Evidence in Transplantation at the Royal College of Surgeons of England. Neil is currently a specialist registrar in General Surgery in the Eastern Deanery.

Neil has a keen interest in teaching both medical students and junior doctors, and was an anatomy demonstrator at St Andrews University. In addition, he is peer reviewer for the journal *Transplantation* and has published extensively in the field of Transplant Surgery. Outside medicine, Neil's main interests are in sport. He is a keen golfer and footballer. He played university first-team football at St Andrews and gained a Cambridge Blue in golf in 2000.

General Surgery

QUESTIONS

1.1 Which of the following conditions is NOT associated with dysphagia?
a Myasthenia gravis
b Achalasia
c Plummer-Vinson syndrome
d Hypothyroidism
e Thoracic aortic aneurysm

1.2 A 75-year-old man presents to the gastroenterology clinic with a three-month history of progressive dysphagia and a hoarse voice. Which of the following investigations would you carry out first?
a Chest X-ray
b Oesophagoscopy
c Barium swallow
d CT scan of the thorax and abdomen
e Endoscopic ultrasound

1.3 A three-week-old male infant presents to A&E with non-bilious projectile vomiting and failure to thrive. The most likely diagnosis is:
a Duodenal atresia
b Overfeeding
c Gastroenteritis
d Intracranial birth injury
e Congenital hypertrophic pyloric stenosis

1.4   *Helicobacter pylori* is a:
   a   Gram-positive, non-motile coccus
   b   Gram-positive, motile coccus
   c   Gram-negative, motile rod
   d   Gram-negative, non-motile rod
   e   Spirochaete

1.5   An 82-year-old woman presents to A&E with a short history of sudden-onset, severe epigastric pain that is aggravated by movement. She has a long history of osteoarthritis, for which she takes regular Voltarol. The most likely diagnosis is:
   a   Perforated appendicitis
   b   Acute pancreatitis
   c   Perforated peptic ulcer
   d   Myocardial infarction
   e   Acute cholecystitis

1.6   Which of the following conditions is NOT associated with gastrointestinal haemorrhage?
   a   Peptic ulcer disease
   b   Meckel's diverticulum
   c   Angiodysplasia
   d   Mallory-Weiss syndrome
   e   Pernicious anaemia

1.7   Risk factors for gastric carcinoma do NOT include:
   a   Previous gastric surgery
   b   Chronic peptic ulcer disease
   c   Blood group B
   d   Smoking
   e   Low socio-economic status

1.8   Which of the following symptoms generally occurs first in small-bowel obstruction?
   a   Colicky abdominal pain
   b   Vomiting
   c   Absolute constipation
   d   Abdominal distension
   e   Pyrexia

1.9 Which of the following is NOT a luminal cause of bowel obstruction?
a Gallstone
b Faeces
c Intussusception
d Diverticulitis
e Parasitic infection

1.10 An 85-year-old man presents to A&E with acute-onset colicky abdominal pain and has had some passage of altered blood per rectum. On examination, he is shocked, in atrial fibrillation and generally tender on abdominal palpation. The most likely diagnosis is:
a Ischaemic bowel
b Peptic ulcer disease
c Diverticulitis
d Sigmoid volvulus
e Acute appendicitis

1.11 Hirschsprung's disease is produced by abnormal development of the:
a Sympathetic innervation of the proximal bowel
b Parasympathetic innervation of the proximal bowel
c Sympathetic innervation of the distal bowel
d Parasympathetic innervation of the distal bowel
e Cholinergic innervation of the proximal bowel

1.12 Intussusception in children is usually secondary to:
a A polyp
b A carcinoma
c Meckel's diverticulum
d A lymphoma
e No obvious cause

1.13 A 25-year-old male patient presents to his GP with a several-day history of lower-abdominal pain followed by loose motions and fevers. Which of following is the best course of management?

a The patient should be referred to the gastroenterologists for management of Crohn's disease.

b The patient should be reassured and sent home with advice to drink plenty of fluids.

c The patient should be sent home with a course of ciprofloxacin.

d The patient should be referred to the surgeons, as this is likely to be acute appendicitis.

e The patient should be urged to return to the surgery in one week for reassessment.

1.14 A middle-aged woman presents to her GP with a short history of abdominal distension and weight loss, along with an everted umbilicus. The most likely diagnosis is:

a Pancreatic cancer

b Ovarian cancer

c Colon cancer

d Gastric cancer

e Hepatoma

1.15 A 70-year-old woman is admitted to hospital deeply jaundiced. She denies having any abdominal pain but has a history of weight loss and itching. On examination, she is cachexic and has a palpable gall bladder, but her abdomen is otherwise non-tender. The most likely diagnosis is:

a Lymphoma

b Hepatitis

c Cholangitis

d Carcinoma of the head of the pancreas

e Chronic cholecystitis

1.16 Which of the following is NOT associated with constipation?

a Diverticular disease

b Myxoedema

c Dyschezia

d Hirschsprung's disease

e Digitalis

1.17 A 65-year-old male patient presents to the outpatient clinic with a long history of constipation only. Which of the following is the most appropriate investigation for him?
  a Colonoscopy
  b Barium enema
  c CT scan of the abdomen and pelvis
  d Rigid sigmoidoscopy
  e Flexible sigmoidoscopy

1.18 Angiodysplasia commonly affects the:
  a Duodenum
  b Jejunum
  c Caecum
  d Transverse colon
  e Rectum

1.19 Which of the following is only associated with Crohn's disease?
  a Granulomas on microscopy
  b Fistulae
  c Gastrointestinal haemorrhage
  d Strictures
  e Pyoderma gangrenosum

1.20 What percentage of large-bowel tumours are synchronous (multiple)?
  a 1%
  b 2%
  c 5%
  d 10%
  e 15%

1.21 Hereditary non-polyposis colon cancer is likely if:
  a At least four family members have been diagnosed with colon cancer, spanning two generations, with one before the age of 60
  b At least three family members have been diagnosed with colon cancer, spanning two generations, with one before the age of 55
  c At least three family members have been diagnosed with colon cancer, spanning two generations, with one before the age of 60
  d At least four family members have been diagnosed with colon cancer, spanning two generations, with one before the age of 50
  e At least three family members have been diagnosed with colon cancer, spanning two generations, with one before the age of 50

1.22 In familial adenomatous polyposis (FAP), the polyps first appear in:
a Infancy
b Adolescence
c Early adulthood
d Middle age
e Old age

1.23 What is the five-year survival for a Dukes' A adenocarcinoma of the colon?
a 65%
b 70%
c 80%
d 90%
e 100%

1.24 What is the most common cause of bright-red rectal bleeding?
a Anal fissure
b Diverticular disease
c Trauma
d Haemorrhoids
e Tumours of the colon and rectum

1.25 Acute perianal pain is associated with:
a Anal fissure
b Thrombosed haemorrhoids
c Perianal abscess
d Proctalgia fugax
e All of the above

1.26 Which of the following statements is true regarding anal fistulae?
a Goodsall's rule states that anterior anal fistulae open radially (directly), whereas posterior anal fistulae open into the midline.
b Goodsall's rule states that anterior anal fistulae open into the midline, whereas posterior anal fistulae open radially.
c Goodsall's rule states that anterior anal fistulae open laterally, whereas posterior anal fistulae open into the midline.
d Goodsall's rule states that anterior anal fistulae open into the midline, whereas posterior anal fistulae open laterally.
e Goodsall's rule states that both anterior and posterior anal fistulae open into the midline.

1.27 Posterior midline anal fissures occur in about:
   a 70% men and 90% women
   b 60% men and 60% women
   c 90% men and 10% women
   d 90% men and 70% women
   e 80% men and 50% women

1.28 Which of the following statements is true regarding groin hernias?
   a Femoral hernias occur less commonly in women than in men.
   b An indirect inguinal hernia can be felt to lie below and medial to the pubic tubercle.
   c The neck of a femoral hernia always lies below and medial to the pubic tubercle.
   d Congenital inguinal hernias obliterate spontaneously.
   e 60% of inguinal hernias occur on the right side, 20% occur on the left and 20% are bilateral.

1.29 Which of the following statements is true regarding paralytic ileus?
   a Colicky abdominal pain is a prominent feature.
   b A completely silent abdomen is diagnostic of paralytic ileus.
   c A plain X-ray of the abdomen will always show localised loops of distended small bowel.
   d Paralytic ileus never lasts more than three days post-operatively.
   e Paralytic ileus and mechanical obstruction cannot coexist.

1.30 Which of the following statements is true regarding gallstones?
   a Diabetes is not a risk factor for gallstone disease.
   b Gallstones are always symptomatic.
   c Gallstones are about half as common in men.
   d Urgent laparoscopic cholecystectomy for acute gallstone disease should be carried out within the first three to four weeks.
   e A common bile duct stone of up to 5 mm in size can pass spontaneously.

1.31 In proven cases of obstructive jaundice secondary to gallstones, which of the following would you organise?
a Ultrasound scan of the abdomen
b Magnetic resonance cholangiopancreatography (MRCP)
c Computed tomography of the abdomen (CT)
d Endoscopic retrograde cholangiopancreatography (ERCP)
e Percutaneous transhepatic cholangiography (PTC)

1.32 Which of the following organisms is responsible for hydatid disease?
a *Clonorchis sinensis*
b *Echinococcus granulosus*
c *Fasciola hepatica*
d *Strongyloides stercoralis*
e *Calodium hepaticum*

1.33 Which of the following statements is true regarding acute pancreatitis?
a Urinary amylase returns to normal within two to three days.
b Ultrasound can always confirm pancreatic inflammation.
c The presence of four or more Glasgow criteria indicate a severe attack of acute pancreatitis.
d Early ERCP is indicated in severe gallstone pancreatitis.
e There is no evidence that nasojejunal feeding is superior to TPN in the supportive management of acute pancreatitis.

1.34 Which of the following statements is true regarding pancreatic carcinoma?
a Microscopically, these tumours are most commonly undifferentiated.
b The incidence is reducing.
c Painful progressive jaundice is the classical presentation.
d CT scanning may demonstrate the tumour mass and facilitate fine-needle biopsy.
e The prognosis is favourable following surgical resection and chemotherapy.

1.35 Which of the following statements is true regarding chronic pancreatitis?
  a Diabetes is rare.
  b Serum amylase is always high during attacks of abdominal pain.
  c Abdominal X-ray may show evidence of calcification along the pancreatic duct.
  d Surgery is only an option if attacks are very frequent.
  e It is always possible to distinguish between chronic pancreatitis and pancreatic carcinoma.

1.36 Six months after anterior resection for a Dukes' C adenocarcinoma of the rectum, a 70-year-old man presents in clinic with a markedly elevated carcinoembryonic antigen (CEA). Which of the following statements is correct?
  a The CEA should be repeated in three months, as it can be elevated post-op.
  b There is likely to be tumour recurrence.
  c A staging laparotomy must be performed.
  d The initial surgical resection was inadequate.
  e Metastasis to the liver is unlikely.

1.37 A 59-year-old woman presents with central colicky abdominal pain that is associated with vomiting and abdominal distention. She last opened her bowels two days ago. On examination, there is a midline laparotomy scar and the abdomen is mildly tender and distended. The rectum is empty on digital rectal examination. The abdominal X-ray is shown (*see* Figure 1). The most likely cause of her symptoms is:
  a Ischaemic bowel
  b Adhesions
  c Sigmoid volvulus
  d Hypothyroidism
  e Constipation

1.38 Which of the following statements is true regarding acute appendicitis?
  a Anorexia is uncommon.
  b Pain starts in the right iliac fossa.
  c Vomiting often precedes pain.
  d It may be caused by obstruction of the appendiceal lumen by a faecolith.
  e Morphine should be avoided until a diagnosis is made.

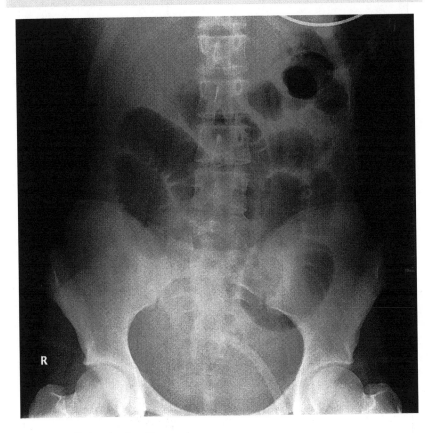

FIGURE 1 Abdominal radiograph

1.39 The most common presentation of a caecal (i.e. right-sided) tumour is with:
  a A palpable mass within the right iliac fossa
  b Iron-deficiency anaemia
  c Change in bowel habits
  d Per rectal bleeding
  e Localised perforation

1.40 Which of the following is associated with an increased incidence of malignancy?
  a Diverticulosis
  b Melanosis coli
  c Irritable bowel syndrome
  d Crohn's disease
  e Duodenal ulcers

1.41 Which of the following statements is true regarding Meckel's diverticula?
a They are rare.
b They are false diverticula.
c They are usually symptomatic.
d They may contain ectopic pancreatic mucosa.
e Bleeding is typically painful.

1.42 A 52-year-old man presents to his GP with a six-month history of episodes of painless per rectal bleeding and pruritus ani. The blood is bright red and often drips into the toilet bowel after the patient strains to open his bowels. The most likely diagnosis is:
a Anal fissure
b Diverticulitis
c Ulcerative colitis
d Colonic polyps
e Haemorrhoids

1.43 A 57-year-old post-menopausal woman presents to her GP with a haemoglobin of 9.7 g/dL, an MCV of 70 and a serum ferritin of 8 μmg/L. She is asymptomatic, and abdominal examination, including rectal examination, is unremarkable. The most appropriate next step is:
a Reassure her and repeat blood tests in six months.
b Send bloods for coeliac serology.
c Refer her for genetic screening.
d Prescribe iron tablets and discharge her.
e CT scan the abdomen and pelvis.

1.44 A 25-year-old male Mediterranean lorry driver presents to A&E with a 2 cm by 3 cm fluctuant, tender, hot lump at the natal cleft. The most likely diagnosis is:
a Perianal abscess
b Pyogenic granuloma
c Pilonidal sinus
d Fistula-in-ano
e Pilonidal abscess

1.45 The micro-organism most commonly implicated in acute cholecystitis is:
a *Klebsiella pneumoniae*
b *Enterobacter* sp.
c *Escherichia coli*
d *Proteus* sp.
e *Enterococcus* sp.

1.46 A 35-year-old woman presents to her GP with a five-week history of pain on defecation and bright red rectal bleeding. On examination, a sentinel pile is noted posteriorly; however, digital rectal examination is precluded due to pain. The most appropriate next step is:
a Ice and bed rest
b Lateral sphincterotomy
c Flexible sigmoidoscopy
d Injection with 5% phenol in almond oil
e Topical GTN cream

1.47 An 80-year-old woman presents to A&E with a two-day history of generalised abdominal pain, absolute constipation and abdominal distension. On examination, she is apyrexial, blood pressure is 110/90 mmHg and heart rate is 90 bpm. The abdomen is grossly distended, mildly tender and tympanic to percussion. Digital rectal examination reveals an empty rectum. The plain abdominal X-ray is shown below (*see* Figure 2). The most appropriate next step is:
a Laparotomy
b Observe
c Rigid/flexible sigmoidoscopy
d Urgent CT scan of the abdomen/pelvis
e Repeat abdominal X-ray

1.48 Which of the following statements is true regarding the midgut?
a Pain is referred to the epigastrium.
b Its blood supply is derived from the inferior mesenteric artery.
c It extends from the duodenal papilla to the splenic flexure.
d Structures include the liver.
e During embryological development, the midgut undergoes a 270° clockwise rotation before returning to the abdominal cavity.

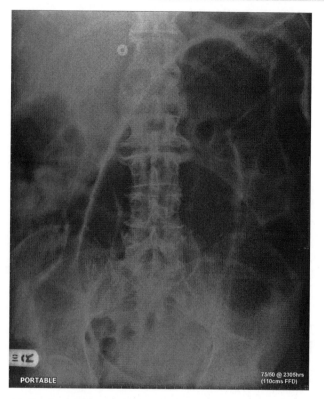

FIGURE 2 Abdominal radiograph

1.49 Which of the following have some prognostic value in acute pancreatitis?
a Serum amylase >1000 U/L
b White cell count >15 000/mm³
c AST >100 U/L
d Age >50 years
e Serum LDH >500 U/L

1.50 A 27-year-old woman presents to A&E with a one-day history of right iliac fossa pain, nausea and anorexia. Abdominal examination reveals marked tenderness in the right iliac fossa and soft stool in the rectum on digital rectal examination. The following are likely to aid diagnosis, EXCEPT:
a Urinalysis
b Urinary β-hCG
c Abdominal X-ray
d Ultrasound scan of the pelvis
e Laparoscopy

1.51 The following conditions may give rise to an elevated serum amylase, EXCEPT:
a Renal failure
b Perforated duodenal ulcer
c Dissecting aortic aneurysm
d Ectopic pregnancy
e Sigmoid diverticula

1.52 Which of the following statements is true regarding the extra-intestinal manifestations of inflammatory bowel disease (IBD)?
a Primary sclerosing cholangitis is associated with Crohn's disease.
b Pyogenic gangrenosum is rarely seen near the site of stomas.
c Uveitis and episcleritis are the most common extra-intestinal manifestations.
d There is an association between ankylosing spondylitis and HLA-B23.
e Erythema nodosum usually occurs on the flexor surfaces of the limbs.

1.53 A 40-year-old man is out at dinner, and over the course of the evening he has consumed a fair amount of alcohol. He vomits forcefully and thereafter complains of sudden onset of severe chest pain. When seen in A&E, he is shocked, subcutaneous emphysema is noted in the neck and guarding is demonstrated within the epigastrium. The most likely diagnosis is:
a Mallory-Weiss tear
b Myocardial infarction
c Boerhaave's syndrome
d Acute pancreatitis
e Perforated peptic ulcer

1.54 Which of the following statements is true regarding oesophageal cancer?
a Smoking and alcohol consumption are risk factors for adenocarcinoma.
b Adenocarcinoma usually affects the upper third of the oesophagus.
c Squamous cell carcinoma is the most common type in developed countries.
d It has a good prognosis.
e Voice hoarseness is a feature of advanced disease.

1.55 A 35-year-old obese man presents to his GP with a three-week history of dyspepsia that is worse on eating and associated with acid brash. In addition, he experiences odynophagia with hot drinks. He denies any symptoms of dysphagia or weight loss. He is a smoker and drinks 35 units of alcohol a week. Examination is unremarkable. The most likely diagnosis is:

a Gastro-oesophageal reflux disease (GORD)
b Gastric ulcer
c Duodenal ulcer
d Oesophageal cancer
e Oesophageal stricture

1.56 A 52-year-old man presents in clinic with fresh rectal bleeding. This is not associated with any pain, weight loss or change in bowel habit. The blood is bright red and not mixed in with the stool. He has no family history of bowel cancer. Clinical examination demonstrates third degree haemorrhoids on proctoscopy only. The most appropriate next step is:

a Abdominal X-ray
b Colonoscopy
c Faecal occult blood testing
d Flexible sigmoidoscopy
e Haemorrhoidectomy

1.57 A 53-year-old obese woman presents in clinic with a one-month history of a non-tender reducible lump in the periumbilical region. She denies any symptoms of vomiting, abdominal pain, abdominal distension or absolute constipation, and is otherwise fit. Examination reveals a plum-sized reducible lump at the umbilicus, which is reducible and transmits a cough impulse. The most appropriate next step is:

a Abdominal X-ray to exclude obstruction
b Ultrasound scan
c CT scan of the abdomen
d Emergency surgical repair
e Elective surgical repair

1.58 Which of the following statements is true regarding colonic polyps?
   a Hyperplastic polyps have malignant potential.
   b Large adenomatous polyp size is associated with greater malignant potential.
   c Villous adenomas typically are found in the ascending colon.
   d Hypokalaemia is a recognised complication of metaplastic polyps.
   e Adenomatous polyps are more common than hyperplastic polyps.

1.59 A 43-year-old woman presents with a two-day history of sudden-onset excruciating perianal pain. She has a medical history of atrial fibrillation and is on warfarin. On examination, a bluish-purple tender lump is found in the perianal region. Which of the following would not form part of the patient's immediate management?
   a Surgical excision
   b Oral analgesia
   c Laxatives
   d Topical lignocaine ointment
   e Cold pack to perianal region

1.60 A two-day-old neonate is reviewed, as his mother is concerned that he has not passed meconium and he has bilious vomiting. On examination, the abdomen is distended and the anal sphincter is tight. Abdominal X-ray demonstrates distended large bowel. The most likely diagnosis is:
   a Duodenal atresia
   b Hypertrophic pyloric stenosis
   c Hirschsprung's disease
   d Toxic megacolon
   e Imperforate anus

1.61 Which of the following statements is true regarding the NHS Bowel Cancer Screening Programme?
   a Screening is offered every five years.
   b Only men are included in the programme.
   c It includes those between the ages of 59 and 70 years.
   d Screening involves a blood test for CEA and faecal occult blood testing (FOBT).
   e The sensitivity of unrehydrated FOBT for colorectal cancer is approximately 55–57%.

1.62 A 75-year-old woman presents with a one-day history of a painful lump in the left groin with associated nausea and vomiting. On examination, she has a tender, irreducible, tense egg-sized lump in the groin. It does not transmit a cough impulse and has overlying skin erythema. Bowel sounds cannot be auscultated. The most likely diagnosis is:
   a Incarcerated inguinal hernia
   b Saphenovarix
   c Strangulated femoral hernia
   d Groin abscess
   e Inguinal lymphadenopathy

1.63 A 40-year-old man is out binge drinking. He wretches and vomits multiple times. He then experiences an episode of haematemesis. He is otherwise fit and well. On examination in A&E, his blood pressure is 110/80 mmHg, his heart rate is 80 bpm and abdominal examination is unremarkable. The most likely diagnosis is:
   a Boerhaave's syndrome
   b Mallory-Weiss tear
   c Oesophageal varices
   d Bleeding duodenal ulcer
   e Oesophagitis

1.64 In intestinal ischaemia, the artery most commonly affected is the:
   a Coeliac trunk
   b Renal artery
   c Superior mesenteric artery
   d Inferior mesenteric artery
   e Internal iliac artery

1.65 Which of the following statements is true regarding hiatus hernias?
   a They are more common in men.
   b Sliding hernias usually require surgery.
   c They are best imaged with oesophagogastroduodenoscopy.
   d Dysphagia is a common symptom of rolling hernias.
   e Rolling hernias are more common than sliding hernias.

1.66 A 35-year-old presents with a six-month history of episodes of sudden-onset sharp anal pain that lasts for a few seconds; this typically occurs at night and resolves spontaneously. She has a medical history of irritable bowel syndrome, for which she takes Buscopan as required. Digital rectal examination, proctoscopy and rigid sigmoidoscopy are normal. The most likely diagnosis is:
a Pruritus ani
b Proctalgia fugax
c Psychosomatic
d Perianal abscess
e Chronic anal fissure

1.67 A sciatic hernia passes through:
a The lesser sciatic foramen
b The greater sciatic foramen
c The obturator canal
d The arcuate line into the lateral border of the posterior rectus sheath
e The inferior lumbar triangle

1.68 Acquired hiatal hernias can be divided into:
a 10% rolling, 90% sliding
b 90% rolling, 10% sliding
c 50% rolling, 50% sliding
d 70% rolling, 30% sliding
e 30% rolling, 70% sliding

1.69 Which of the following statements is true of cholangiocarcinoma?
a The incidence is decreasing.
b A curative resection must always be attempted.
c Palliation is often achieved by endoluminal stenting at ERCP.
d A Whipple's procedure is possible if the tumour affects the proximal common bile duct.
e It usually presents with painful jaundice.

1.70 Which of the following statements is true of gastrointestinal stromal tumours (GISTs)?
a They are more common in men than in women.
b The pathogenesis is a spontaneous mutation in the K-ras gene.
c Chemotherapy is the treatment of choice.
d They may be malignant or benign.
e They typically affect young adults.

1.71 Which of the following statements is NOT true of carcinoid tumours?
a They are amine precursor uptake and decarboxylation tumours.
b 90% are associated with MEN type 1.
c They are commonly found in the appendix.
d Urinary 5-HIAA levels are usually raised.
e Metastasis occurs to regional lymph nodes and the liver.

1.72 Which of the following strategies is NOT employed in the management of bleeding oesophageal varices?
a Endoscopic sclerotherapy
b Endoscopic variceal band ligation
c Intravenous vasopressin
d Transjugular intrahepatic portosystemic shunt
e Intravenous β-blockers

1.73 Which of the following statements is true after a splenectomy?
a The platelet count falls.
b There is no need for post-operative antibiotics.
c Gastric dilatation may follow unless a nasogastric tube is placed perioperatively.
d Prophylactic immunisations must always be given within 24 hours of the operation.
e Adults need lifelong antibiotic prophylaxis.

1.74 Which of the following statements is true regarding pharyngeal pouch?
a It is a mucosal protrusion between the two parts of the superior pharyngeal constrictor.
b It develops anteriorly.
c It is a pulsion diverticulum.
d It is more common in young women.
e It is always palpable.

1.75 Which of the following statements is true regarding carcinoma of the gall bladder?
a It is associated with gallstones in 10% of cases.
b It is more common in men.
c It is adenocarcinoma in 90% of cases.
d It can never be managed operatively.
e It carries a good prognosis.

1.76 Which of the following statements is true regarding pelvic abscesses?
a They are common following elective anterior resections.
b They occur between the rectum and the bladder in women.
c They are always managed with antimicrobials.
d They may present with diarrhoea.
e They are encouraged to discharge through the vagina.

ANSWERS

1.1 The correct answer is D.

Dysphagia (difficulty in swallowing food or liquid) is associated with neurological conditions such as myaesthenia gravis and bulbar palsy or with achalasia where there is failure of oesophageal peristalsis and relaxation of the lower oesophageal sphincter. In addition, oesophageal webs associated with iron-deficiency anaemia can also present with dysphagia.

1.2 The correct answer is B.

The history is suggestive of oesophageal carcinoma; therefore, an oesophagoscopy should be the first investigation performed.

1.3 The correct answer is E.

This is a classical presentation of congenital hypertrophic pyloric stenosis, which affects infants, usually male, under 12 weeks of age (most commonly seen at four weeks after birth). The vomitus is projectile and does not contain bile; weight loss and dehydration are prominent features. Ultrasound is the imaging modality of choice.

1.4 The correct answer is C.

Helicobacter pylori is a spiral-shaped, Gram-negative, motile rod.

1.5 The correct answer is C.

The most likely diagnosis in this age group is perforated peptic ulcer, particularly in those patients who have been on long-term non-steroidal anti-inflammatory drugs for arthritis.

1.6 The correct answer is E.

Pernicious anaemia is not known to be associated with gastrointestinal bleeding.

1.7 The correct answer is C.

Blood group A is associated with gastric carcinoma.

1.8 The correct answer is A.

Usually the patient complains of colicky periumbilical pain first. Vomiting occurs early in high obstruction. Distension is more marked in distal small-bowel or large- bowel obstruction. Pyrexia is a clinical sign, not a symptom, and is associated with strangulated bowel.

1.9 The correct answer is D.

Diverticulitis involves inflammation of the colonic wall and is not a luminal cause.

1.10 The correct answer is A.

The patient has ischaemic bowel. Given that the patient is in atrial fibrillation, the most likely cause is a mesenteric emboli arising from the left atrium. Other causes of mesenteric emboli include mural thrombus secondary to myocardial infarction, heart valve vegetations and atheromatous plaques on the aorta. Importantly, shock is common in acute intestinal ischaemia, and the pain described is classically central and often disproportionate to the clinical findings.

1.11 The correct answer is D.

Hirschsprung's disease is caused by the faulty development of the parasympathetic innervation of the distal bowel. There is an absence of ganglion cells in the submucosal plexus of Auerbach and the intermyenteric plexus of Meissner, affecting mainly the rectum. The involved segment is spastic, causing a functional obstruction with gross proximal dilatation of the colon. It can present in the first few days of life with acute large-bowel obstruction.

1.12 The correct answer is E.

In adults and some children, intussusception may be caused by polyps, tumours or Meckel's, but usually there is no obvious cause found in children. It is postulated that the lymphoid tissue in Peyer's patches within the bowel wall undergoes hyperplasia due to an adenovirus. The swollen lymphoid tissue then protrudes into the lumen and acts as a foreign body that is then propelled distally by peristalsis, dragging the bowel behind it.

1.13 The correct answer is D.

This is likely to be acute appendicitis. The pain typically commences as periumbilical colic that then migrates to the right iliac fossa, but often patients cannot localise the pain well and complain of lower abdominal pain. Diarrhoea can occur if the ileum is irritated by the inflamed appendix. Other symptoms include nausea and vomiting, anorexia and constipation. It is important not to dismiss these symptoms as gastroenteritis unless there are compelling features in the history to suggest this.

1.14 The correct answer is B.

Ovarian cancer classically presents insidiously with a history of weight loss and abdominal distension, so this is the most likely diagnosis. A CT scan of the abdomen and pelvis should be organised.

1.15 The correct answer is D.

Carcinoma of the head of the pancreas usually presents with painless jaundice, and classically a non-tender gall bladder can be palpated on examination. An ultrasound scan of the biliary tree followed by a CT scan of the abdomen would be appropriate next line investigations.

1.16 The correct answer is E.

Digitalis is usually associated with diarrhoea rather than with constipation. Dyschezia is rectal stasis due to a faulty bowel habit. Diverticular disease, hypothyroidism and Hirschsprung's disease are all classically associated with constipation.

1.17 The correct answer is B.

Without any other worrying features, a barium enema would be most appropriate, as the most likely diagnosis is diverticular disease. A CT scan would be best if the patient was admitted with a presumptive diagnosis of diverticulitis, as a barium enema in this instance would carry a high risk of iatrogenic large-bowel perforation.

1.18 The correct answer is C.

Angiodysplasia is the term applied to one or more small submucosal vascular malformations. They are usually asymptomatic but can bleed, and they are most commonly found in the caecum and ascending colon.

1.19 The correct answer is A.

This is because there is considerable overlap between Crohn's disease and ulcerative colitis otherwise.

1.20 The correct answer is C.

1.21 The correct answer is E.

1.22 The correct answer is B.

FAP polyps first appear in adolescence, with symptoms of bleeding and diarrhoea starting in the early 20s, so the correct answer is B. Malignant transformation occurs by the age of 40. Treatment entails a panproctocolectomy and formation of an ileoanal pouch.

1.23 The correct answer is D.

Five-year survival with Dukes' B, where the disease is confined to the bowel wall, is around 65%. With Dukes' C, where there are lymph node metastases, the five year survival is around 30%.

1.24 The correct answer is D.

Although all of these conditions can present with rectal bleeding, the most common cause is haemorrhoids, so the correct answer is D.

1.25 The correct answer is E.

All of the conditions listed can account for severe perianal pain. Other possible conditions include tumours of the anal canal and perianal haematoma.

1.26 The correct answer is A.

1.27 The correct answer is D.

1.28 The correct answer is E.

Femoral hernias occur more commonly in women than in men. An indirect hernia can be felt to lie above and medial to the pubic tubercle, whereas a femoral hernia lies below and lateral to this landmark. Congenital inguinal hernias do not obliterate spontaneously and require surgical repair.

1.29 The correct answer is B.

The symptoms of paralytic ileus include abdominal distension, absolute constipation and effortless vomiting. Colicky abdominal pain is not usually present. On examination, an absolutely silent abdomen usually confirms the diagnosis. X-rays will show gas distributed throughout the small and large bowel. This condition can last longer than three to four days, but persisting symptoms should be regarded as suspicious of alternative diagnoses, including mechanical bowel obstruction or even an anastomotic leak.

1.30 The correct answer is C.

Diabetes is associated with an increased prevalence of gallstones. Gallstones are most commonly asymptomatic. A laparoscopic cholecystectomy following an episode of acute cholecystitis is usually undertaken about six weeks after resolution of symptoms. Common bile duct stones up to 3 mm can pass spontaneously.

1.31 The correct answer is D.

ERCP is indicated, as it is both diagnostic and therapeutic.

1.32 The correct answer is B.

1.33 The correct answer is D.

Urinary amylase is elevated for a longer period than serum amylase and is useful in patients who present late. Ultrasound is the first-line investigation in acute pancreatitis because it can demonstrate gallstones and intrahepatic or extrahepatic duct dilatation. Three or more Glasgow criteria predict a severe attack. There is good evidence that nasojejunal feeding may be superior to TPN, in the absence of an ileus. This is largely due to improved maintenance of gut mucosal integrity with nasojejunal feeding, which thereby reduces septic complications.

1.34 The correct answer is D.

Microscopically, most tumours are adenocarcinomas; the rest are either acinar cell carcinomas or cystadenocarcinomas. The incidence is increasing rather than reducing, particularly in the US. Painless progressive jaundice is the classical presentation. The prognosis is poor, and curative surgical resection is only appropriate in approximately 15% of cases.

1.35 The correct answer is C.

Diabetes is common due to β-cell damage within the pancreas. Serum amylase can rise during attacks, but can also be normal if there is insufficient remaining pancreatic tissue to effect a rise. Surgery, either a partial or complete pancreatectomy, can be carried out in extreme cases. However, the use of surgery is not determined by the frequency of attacks alone. It can be difficult to distinguish between pancreatic carcinoma and chronic pancreatitis on imaging alone.

1.36 The correct answer is B.

CEA is a useful indicator of tumour recurrence. CEA usually returns to normal levels within one to two months post-curative resection. It is often markedly elevated in patients with liver metastases.

1.37 The correct answer is B.

The patient has small-bowel obstruction (SBO). SBO classically presents with colicky, central abdominal pain; vomiting (this usually occurs early and may be faeculent); abdominal distension; and absolute constipation (this often occurs late). On examination, there is abdominal distension and high-pitched bowel sounds. In the UK, the most common causes are groin hernia and adhesions from previous surgery.

1.38 The correct answer is D.

The classic presentation is with a history of anorexia and with periumbilical pain that migrates to the right iliac fossa. When vomiting occurs, it nearly always follows the onset of pain. Vomiting that precedes pain is suggestive of intestinal obstruction, and the diagnosis of appendicitis should be reconsidered. Obstruction of the appendiceal lumen by a faecolith or lymphoid follicle hyperplasia is thought to precipitate appendicitis.

1.39 The correct answer is B.

Caecal tumours account for approximately 20% of all large-bowel cancers. They may present with a right iliac fossa mass, small-bowel obstruction and perforation. Less commonly, they present with acute appendicitis. Left-sided colon and rectal cancers typically present with an alteration in bowel habits and bleeding per rectum.

1.40 The correct answer is D.

Crohn's disease is associated with an increased risk of small-bowel adenocarcinoma.

1.41 The correct answer is D.

Meckel's diverticula are the most common congenital disorder of the small bowel, and they occur due to failure of obliteration of the vitellointestinal duct. They are an example of a true diverticulum, as all layers of the bowel wall are involved. Although approximately half of all Meckel's diverticula contain ectopic mucosa (e.g. gastric, pancreatic mucosa), they are usually asymptomatic. Heterotopic gastric mucosa may give rise to painless bleeding. Remember the rule of '2s': Meckel's diverticula affect 2% of the population, typically exist 2 feet (61 cm) from the ileocaecal valve and are approximately 2 inches (5 cm) in diameter.

1.42 The correct answer is E.

Haemorrhoids are common, affecting 50% of those over the age of 50 years (peak incidence is 45–65 years). Presentation is commonly with fresh rectal bleeding, pruritus ani, prolapse and pain (if thrombosed).

1.43 The correct answer is B.

The most common cause of iron-deficiency anaemia (IDA) in adult men and post-menopausal women is blood loss from the gastrointestinal tract. According to the British Society of Gastroenterology (BSG) guidelines, all patients in this group should have urinalysis for haematuria to exclude renal tract malignancy, coeliac serology and OGD and colonoscopy, if the latter is negative. IDA should also be corrected with iron therapy or blood transfusion in selected cases.

1.44 The correct answer is E.

Pilonidal abscesses arise from a pilonidal sinus/cyst. Pilonidal disease most commonly affects young adult men. Other risk factors include hirsutism and occupations that involve a lot of sitting, and there is often a family history. Management is surgical incision and drainage of the abscess, with subsequent excision of the sinus.

1.45 The correct answer is C.

All of the aforementioned organisms are, however, implicated in acute cholecystitis and ascending cholangitis.

1.46 The correct answer is E.

The patient has an anal fissure. The majority of anal fissures will heal spontaneously. Topical GTN relaxes the internal anal sphincter, reducing the anal resting pressure, thus facilitating healing. Surgical intervention, i.e. lateral sphincterotomy, is indicated if conservative treatment fails. Flexible sigmoidoscopy is unlikely to be tolerated due to pain and is not necessary. Ice and bed rest are useful in the management of thrombosed haemorrhoids. Injection with 5% phenol in almond oil is used in the management of haemorrhoids, not in the management of anal fissures.

1.47 The correct answer is C.

The patient has a sigmoid volvulus. Classic features of an inverted U-shaped bowel loop ('coffee-bean' sign) and absence of gas within the rectum are demonstrated on the abdominal radiograph. The sigmoid colon is the most common site of colonic volvulus. Sigmoidoscopy is both diagnostic and therapeutic, and the majority will settle with conservative treatment. Due to the high incidence of recurrence, surgery may be advocated electively. Emergency surgery is indicated if there is any suspicion of bowel ischaemia.

1.48 The correct answer is C.

Pain from the midgut is referred to the umbilical region. The blood supply of the midgut is from the superior mesenteric artery. Structures of the midgut include the distal duodenum, jejunum, ileum, appendix, ascending colon and majority of the transverse colon. During embryological development, the midgut undergoes a 270° anticlockwise rotation before and during its return to the abdominal cavity.

1.49 The correct answer is B.

Serum amylase (a pancreatic enzyme) is released and reaches peak levels early (2–12 hours following onset of symptoms) in an acute attack, declining over 3–4 days. Levels therefore need to be interpreted with respect to onset of symptoms. Prognostic features that predict disease severity in acute pancreatitis include clinical impression of severity, pleural effusion on chest X-ray, obesity, or APACHE II >8 on initial assessment. Other prognostic indices include C-reactive protein (CRP) >150 mg/L, modified Glasgow score >3, or persisting organ failure after 48 hours in hospital. The modified Glasgow score includes age >55 years, white cell count >15 × 10^9/L, urea >16 mmol/L, glucose >10 mmol/L, pO$_2$ <8 kPa (60 mmHg), albumin <32 g/L, calcium <2 mmol/L, LDH >600 U/L, and AST/ALT >200 U/L.

1.50 The correct answer is C.

Acute appendicitis is a clinical diagnosis. Other causes of right iliac fossa pain include gynaecological causes (e.g. ectopic pregnancy, ruptured ovarian cysts, torsion of the fallopian tubes), urological causes (e.g. ureteric colic, urinary tract infection) and other gastrointestinal causes. A pregnancy test should be performed in all pre-menopausal women with an acute abdomen. Urinalysis is useful for excluding urinary tract infection and haematuria (seen in renal colic). Ultrasound scan and laparoscopy are useful for excluding gynaecological pathology. Ultrasound is not very sensitive for diagnosing acute appendicitis.

1.51 The correct answer is E.

In a normal healthy individual, the majority of serum amylase is derived from the pancreas and salivary glands. However, other organs also produce and secrete amylase and can give rise to mild to moderate increases in serum amylase. These organs include the fallopian tubes, testes, lungs, thyroid and tonsils, and certain cancers can also effect a rise. Amylase is excreted by the kidneys, and acute or chronic renal failure can lead to increases in serum amylase levels. An aortic dissection may compromise the blood supply to the pancreas, leading to pancreatic damage and a subsequent rise in serum amylase.

1.52 The correct answer is C.

Primary sclerosing cholangitis is associated with ulcerative colitis (UC). Pyogenic gangrenosum usually occurs at sites of previous trauma, with the commonest sites being the shins and adjacent to stomas. Uveitis is more common with UC, and episcleritis is more common with Crohn's disease. An association is seen with HLA B-27 in the majority of patients with sacroiliitis and ankylosing spondylitis, which is common in Crohn's disease. Erythema nodosum commonly affects the extensor surfaces, particularly on the lower limbs, and it is associated with active disease, i.e. colitis.

1.53 The correct answer is C.

Boerhaave's syndrome is spontaneous perforation of the oesophagus, typically of the lower third. This leads to mediastinitis due to the introduction of gastrointestinal contents into the mediastinum. Complications include subcutaneous emphysema, pneumothorax, pleural effusion, sepsis and arrhythmias. Diagnosis is made on clinical findings and with a contrast swallow study.

1.54 The correct answer is E.

Smoking and alcohol consumption are risk factors for squamous cell carcinoma of the oesophagus. Adenocarcinoma is associated with Barrett's oesophagus. Squamous cell carcinoma usually occurs in the upper two thirds of the oesophagus, with adenocarcinoma affecting the lower third. Squamous cell carcinoma is the most common type of oesophageal cancer worldwide and is endemic in some parts of China and South Africa. Adenocarcinoma is the most common type of oesophageal cancer in developed countries. Oesophageal cancer has a poor prognosis, with a five-year survival rate of 5–30%. Voice hoarseness occurs due to involvement of the recurrent laryngeal nerve and is suggestive of advanced disease. Other features of advanced disease are weight loss, dysphagia (the most common presentation) and regional lymphadenopathy.

1.55 The correct answer is A.

The patient has gastro-oesophageal reflux disease (GORD), which is thought to be caused by incompetence of the lower oesophageal sphincter (LOS). Often the diagnosis is made on the history alone, and the classic description of symptoms is given in the question.

Oesophagogastroscopy (OGD) is often performed to exclude other pathology and is indicated if dyspepsia is associated with chronic gastrointestinal bleeding, weight loss, progressive dysphagia, persistent vomiting, iron-deficiency anaemia or epigastric mass or if a barium meal is suspicious. Most cases of GORD are not investigated; however, in severe cases, oesophageal manometry and 24-hour oesophageal pH recording can be used and will give the diagnosis. Note that proton pump inhibitors (PPIs) should be stopped at least two weeks prior to these investigations. Treatment of GORD includes lifestyle advice, including weight loss; smoking, alcohol and caffeine consumption cessation; raising the head of the bed; and PPIs. Dysphagia is the most common presentation for oesophageal cancer. Duodenal ulcers typically present with anaemia and with epigastric pain that radiates to the back and is often relieved by food. Gastric ulcers have a similar clinical picture to duodenal ulcers; however, the pain is often made worse with food. Oesophageal strictures typically produce dysphagia.

1.56 The correct answer is D.

Although the most likely cause of the bleeding is haemorrhoids, any patient >40 years old requires investigation. Flexible sigmoidoscopy is the investigation of choice in this case. Abdominal X-ray is of no value for rectal bleeding. Faecal occult blood has a 20% false-negative rate for colon cancer. If there is a microcytic anaemia, OGD and colonoscopy are indicated. Haemorrhoidectomy may be performed once other causes are excluded.

1.57 The correct answer is E.

The patient has a paraumbilical hernia. Paraumbilical hernias are approximately five times more common in women and typically occur in middle age. Risk factors include obesity, ascites, multiparity and intra-abdominal malignancy. Elective surgical repair is advocated in adults due to the risk of strangulation or incarceration. Evidence of obstruction or strangulation warrants emergent surgical repair. Usually the diagnosis of a hernia is made clinically and imaging is not required. Ultrasound may be useful to assess for the presence of a hernia if the diagnosis is unclear. CT scan of the abdomen may be useful for complex or elusive hernias.

1.58 The correct answer is B.

Colonic polyps may be categorised as hyperplastic or adenomatous. Hyperplastic or metaplastic polyps account for approximately 90% of all colonic epithelial polyps and do not have any malignant potential. Adenomatous polyps may be further categorised as tubular (most common; may be sessile or pedunculated), villous or tubulovillous. Villous adenomas most frequently affect the rectum and are more likely to be symptomatic; they most commonly cause rectal bleeding and they can also produce symptoms of copious mucus discharge (leading to hypokalaemia).

1.59 The correct answer is A.

The patient has a thrombosed external haemorrhoid. If the patient presents within 48 to 72 hours of onset of symptoms, surgical excision of the haemorrhoid is beneficial (in terms of time till symptom relief, recurrence and reduction in skin tag formation). However, anticoagulation is a contraindication to surgery. The patient should therefore be managed conservatively with bed rest, ice, analgesia and stool softeners. As the thrombus organises, pain reduces and typically starts to decline after 72 hours, but not before reaching a crescendo.

1.60 The correct answer is C.

The patient has Hirschsprung's disease. Hirschsprung's disease has a spectrum of presentation, dependent on age. Neonates typically present with delayed passage of meconium, abdominal distension and bilious vomiting; children of a few months of age may present with chronic constipation and failure to thrive. Rectal biopsy will confirm the diagnosis, and it demonstrates aganglionosis of the Meissner's (submucosal) and/or Auerbach's (myenteric) plexuses and hypertrophy of the nerve fibres. Anal manometry will show absence of internal and sphincter relaxation. In hypertrophic pyloric stenosis, the vomiting is typically non-bilious. Duodenal atresia does not give rise to large-bowel obstruction. With imperforate anus (due to persistence of the anal membrane), there is usually an absence/abnormality of the anal opening.

1.61 The correct answer is E.

The NHS Bowel Cancer Screening Programme was rolled out nationally in 2009. Screening is offered every two years to men and women between the ages of 60 and 69 years (people >70 years may request to be screened). Screening involves faecal occult blood testing (FOBT) from stool samples. A positive faecal occult blood test is investigated further with colonoscopy. Screening with FOBT results in an approximately 16% reduction in mortality from colorectal cancer.

1.62 The correct answer is C.

The patient has a strangulated femoral hernia. Femoral hernias are more common in women, and they are at increased risk of complications of incarceration, obstruction (typically small bowel) and strangulation compared to inguinal hernias. Incarcerated hernias are usually not painful but are typically irreducible. Colicky abdominal pain, abdominal distension, vomiting and absolute constipation suggest obstruction. Shock, peritonitis and increasing pain suggest strangulation; in addition, the hernia is likely to be tense, tender, and irreducible, with an absent cough impulse and skin changes.

1.63 The correct answer is B.

The patient has a Mallory-Weiss tear. This is a longitudinal mucosal tear that typically occurs at the cardia. The majority resolve spontaneously, and endoscopy is diagnostic. Boerhaave's syndrome is spontaneous perforation of the oesophagus, and it does not typically cause haematemesis. In the developed world, alcohol and viral cirrhosis are the most common causes of portal hypertension and oesophageal varices; patients with oesophageal varices will usually display some stigmata of liver disease. With duodenal ulcers, there is usually associated abdominal/epigastric tenderness (which is not common with Mallory-Weiss tears); a history of non-steroidal anti-inflammatory drug (NSAID) use should be elicited. Oesophagitis does not cause haematemesis.

1.64 The correct answer is C.

The superior mesenteric artery (SMA) is most commonly affected in acute intestinal ischaemia. Ischaemia may be due to thrombosis or an embolus. Thrombosis is seen to typically occur at the origin of the SMA, whereas emboli more often lodge at the origin of the middle colic artery. If the SMA is affected, infarction/ischaemia of the bowel occurs, extending from the duodenojejunal flexure to the splenic flexure.

1.65 The correct answer is D.

Hiatus hernias are more common in the Western world, in women and with increasing age. They can be classified as sliding or rolling (paraoesophageal); the majority are sliding. In sliding hernias, the gastro-oesophageal junction and a portion of stomach protrude into the mediastinum through the oesophageal hiatus. In rolling hernias, the fundus of the stomach protrudes above the diaphragm to lie parallel to the oesophagus, while the gastro-oesophageal junction remains below the diaphragm. Hiatus hernias are usually asymptomatic but may give rise to dysphagia (seen with rolling hernias), pain due to incarceration (rare), bleeding (rare) and symptoms of GORD. They are best imaged with a barium meal. Rolling hiatus hernias require surgery due to their increased risk of complications, e.g. incarceration, perforation and strangulation.

1.66 The correct answer is B.

Proctalgia fugax translates from Latin as 'fleeting rectal pain'. No aetiology has been identified; however, it is thought to be due to spasm of the muscles in the rectum and pelvis. It is associated with irritable bowel syndrome. Pruritus ani is itchiness around the anus. With perianal abscesses, signs of localised infection are usually evident. Anal fissures typically give rise to painful defecation and rectal bleeding.

1.67 The correct answer is A.

Gluteal hernias pass through the greater sciatic foramen, obturator hernias pass through the obturator canal and Spigelian hernias develop upwards through the arcuate line into the lateral border of the posterior rectus sheath.

1.68 The correct answer is A.

1.69 The correct answer is C.

The incidence of cholangiocarcinoma is increasing. There are few surgical options once a diagnosis has been reached, as these cases tend to present late. A Whipple's resection may be possible if the tumour is located distally within the common bile duct. Cholangiocarcinoma usually presents with painless progressive jaundice.

1.70 The correct answer is D.

GISTs affect men and women equally. They usually affect those over 40 years of age. The spontaneous mutation arises in the c-kit gene, not the K-ras gene. Wide local excision is recommended.

1.71 The correct answer is B.

Ten per cent of cases are associated with MEN type 1.

1.72 The correct answer is E.

Intravenous β-blockers are useful as prophylaxis against bleeding in oesophageal varices rather than as a manoeuvre to arrest haemorrhaging from oesophageal varices. β-blockers are thought to reduce splanchnic blood flow and thereby lower portal venous pressure.

1.73 The correct answer is C.

The platelet count usually rises following a splenectomy. Prophylactic antibiotics are indicated to minimise the risk of overwhelming post-splenectomy sepsis (OPSS), but in adults they do not need to be taken daily beyond the first two years after a splenectomy. Prophylactic immunisation with pneumococcal, meningococcal and *Haemophilus influenzae* type B vaccines should be given pre-operatively where possible.

1.74 The correct answer is C.

A pharyngeal pouch protrudes between the two parts of the *inferior* pharyngeal constrictor and develops posteriorly. It is more common in older men and may be palpable.

1.75 The correct answer is C.

Carcinoma of the gall bladder is more common in women and is associated with gallstones in 90% of cases. Sometimes small carcinomas are removed inadvertently during elective cholecystectomy for gallstones, but advanced disease is usually not amenable to surgery. Overall, the condition carries a poor prognosis.

1.76 The correct answer is D.

Pelvic abscesses are most common after acute appendicitis and gynaecological infections. These abscesses lie between the bladder and rectum in men and between the uterus and posterior fornix of the vagina anteriorly and the rectum posteriorly in women. Although antimicrobials are used in the treatment of pelvic abscesses, it is generally better to drain the pus through the rectal wall.

Vascular Surgery

QUESTIONS

2.1 Which of the following statements is true regarding primary varicose veins?

a Sapheno-femoral incompetence is more common than sapheno-popliteal incompetence.

b Surgery should not be offered without a prior trial of graded compression stockings.

c Damage to the saphenous nerve during surgery results in foot drop.

d Endovenous laser treatment is only useful for treating sapheno-femoral incompetence.

e They are commonly caused by deep vein thrombosis.

2.2 A 47-year-old man has recently returned to the ward following emergency left common femoral artery embolectomy for an acutely ischaemic left leg. He is on intravenous heparin and has a morphine PCA. You are asked to review him, as he is complaining of severe left-calf pain and swelling. On examination, the calf is swollen and tender. Pedal pulses are palpable. The most appropriate next step is:

a Stop the IV heparin.

b Administer 10 mg intravenous morphine stat and call the pain team.

c Lower the left leg to improve the blood supply.

d Perform left-leg fasciotomy.

e Check the APTT is therapeutic.

2.3 Features of critical limb ischaemia do NOT include:

a Rest pain of greater than two weeks' duration

b Gangrene

c Ulceration

d Toe pressures of <30 mmHg

e A claudication distance of <50 yards (46 metres)

2.4 A 56-year-old unemployed man presents to clinic with a three-month history of right-calf claudication at 8.0 yards (7.2 metres). This is relieved by rest and not associated with rest pain, ulcers or gangrene. He is a heavy smoker and has a medical history of hypertension. Examination reveals a good right femoral, popliteal and dorsalis pedis pulse, with an absent right posterior tibial pulse. Right-leg ABPIs = 0.6. The most appropriate next step is:

a Lower-limb diagnostic angiography

b Right-leg angioplasty

c Optimise medical therapy; advise to 'stop smoking and keep walking'

d Lower-limb CT angiography

e Femoral-distal bypass surgery

2.5 A 63-year-old woman presents with a history over the last few months of episodes of left amaurosis fugax. Examination reveals a left-sided carotid bruit. The most appropriate next step is:

a Carotid endarterectomy

b Carotid angiography

c CT scan brain

d Carotid Doppler ultrasound (duplex)

e MR angiography

2.6 A 79-year-old man presents to A&E with severe epigastric pain that radiates to the back. His peripheries are cold and pale. He has a blood pressure of 60/44 mmHg and a heart rate of 110 bpm. A tender pulsatile mass is palpable within the epigastrium. The most appropriate next step is:

a Urgent CT scan of the abdomen

b Focused assessment with sonography for trauma (FAST) scan in A&E

c Aggressive fluid resuscitation to bring blood pressure to within the normal range

d Theatre

e Transfer to another hospital for emergency endovascular repair

2.7 Which of the following statements is NOT true regarding central venous line insertion?
a Positioning the patient in the Trendelenburg position reduces the risk of air embolus.
b Pneumothorax is more commonly associated with subclavian line insertion.
c A post-insertion chest X-ray should be performed to exclude a pneumothorax.
d Insertion should ideally be performed under ultrasound guidance.
e Cardiac arrhythmia is a recognised complication.

2.8 Which of the following does NOT form part of the management of an acutely ischaemic limb?
a Intramuscular heparin
b Thrombophilia screen
c ECG
d Urinalysis
e Embolectomy

2.9 The most common aetiology of leg ulcers in the United Kingdom is:
a Arterial
b Neuropathic
c Neoplastic
d Venous
e Vasculitic

2.10 The operative mortality associated with ruptured abdominal aortic aneurysm (AAA) repair is:
a <5%
b 10%
c Approximately 50%
d Nearly always fatal
e Dependent on the grade of the surgeon

2.11 Which of the following statements is true regarding venous leg ulcers?
a They commonly lie over the lateral malleolus.
b They usually require skin grafting.
c Four-layer compression bandaging should only be applied if ABPIs are >0.9.
d They rarely heal completely.
e Venous duplex should be performed in all cases.

2.12 A 57-year-old woman presents to A&E with a three-day history of diffuse headache that is worse at night and has become progressively more severe. In addition, she complains of pain in the jaw on chewing. Examination reveals tenderness over the right temporal artery and an afferent pupillary defect. Fundoscopy is normal. ESR is 67 mm/hour. The most appropriate next step is:
a High-dose corticosteroids
b High-dose immunoglobulins
c Urgent temporal artery biopsy
d Intravenous fluorescein angiography
e Referral to an ophthalmologist for assessment of visual acuity

2.13 A 37-year-old woman who is on warfarin and has a known extensive left femoral deep vein thrombosis becomes acutely short of breath, with saturations of 87% on room air. Her blood pressure is 120/76 mmHg and her heart rate is 106 bpm. The most useful first-line investigation would be:
a Repeat lower-limb venous duplex
b CT pulmonary angiogram
c Blood test to ensure INR is within the therapeutic range
d Echocardiogram
e Chest X-ray

2.14 Which of the following is NOT a recognised feature of cardiac tamponade?
a Abolition of the y descent of the jugular venous waveform
b Hypotension
c Raised jugular venous pressure
d Bradycardia
e Pulsus paradoxus

2.15 A 67-year-old man is seen by his GP and is incidentally noted to have a non-tender, expansile and pulsatile mass within his abdomen. His blood pressure is 130/80 mmHg and his heart rate is 70 bpm. The most appropriate next step is:
a Urgent referral to the vascular surgeons
b Ultrasound scan of the abdominal aorta
c Full blood count
d CT scan of the abdomen
e MRA of the abdomen

2.16 Indications for elective AAA repair in men include:
a Age >60 years
b Size >5.5 cm
c Growth rate greater than 0.5 cm per year
d Coexisting popliteal aneurysm
e All of the above

2.17 A 40-year-old woman presents to her GP with varicose veins that have been present since her second pregnancy but have been gradually increasing in size. Clinical examination reveals prominent varicose veins and sapheno-femoral incompetence. Which of the following statements is true?
a Graded compression stockings will provide a permanent cure.
b A venous duplex should be performed.
c She may have coexisting sapheno-popliteal incompetence.
d Venous ulceration is a contraindication for surgery.
e They will spontaneously regress with time.

2.18 A 67-year-old woman presents to A&E with a four-hour history of a cold and painful left leg. She is a smoker and has no other significant co-morbidity. On examination, popliteal and pedal pulses cannot be palpated, and the leg is pale, mottled and cold to the knee, with reduced sensation. An ECG reveals that she is in atrial fibrillation. The most appropriate next step is:
a Left below-knee amputation
b Commence warfarin
c Intravenous amiodarone
d Advise 'stop smoking and keep walking' and optimise vascular risk factors
e Embolectomy

2.19 Four days following her return to England from America, a 29-year-old woman develops a painful, swollen left leg. On examination, the left leg is swollen to the thigh, the calf is tender and all lower-limb pulses are palpable. The most appropriate next step is:
a CT pulmonary angiogram to exclude a pulmonary embolus
b Urgent venous duplex of the left leg
c Therapeutic-dose heparin
d Pelvic ultrasound
e Warfarin

2.20 Which of the following statements is true regarding aneurysms?
   a Approximately 50% of popliteal aneurysms are bilateral.
   b AAAs are more common in Asians.
   c The greatest risk factor for aneurysm formation is diabetes.
   d Splenic artery aneurysms are more common in men.
   e Popliteal aneurysms are more prone to rupture than are AAAs.

2.21 A 56-year-old insulin-dependent diabetic man presents with gangrene of his right big toe. On examination of the right foot, there is wet gangrene of the big toe, with surrounding cellulitis. All lower-limb pulses are palpable, and there is 'glove and stocking' sensory loss. The most appropriate next step is:
   a Intravenous heparin
   b Urgent MRI of the foot
   c Intravenous broad-spectrum antibiotics
   d Hyperbaric oxygen therapy
   e Amputation

2.22 The most common cause of lymphoedema is:
   a Filariasis
   b Milroy's disease
   c Radiotherapy
   d Malignancy
   e Deep vein thrombosis

2.23 A 28-year-old woman presents in clinic complaining of pallor of her fingers when she goes out in the cold. They then become worryingly blue, and then they go red and tingle when she goes indoors. On examination, all upper-limb pulses are palpable, and the hands are warm. The following may be advised in the management of her condition, EXCEPT:
   a Nifedipine
   b Cold avoidance
   c Gloves
   d Iloprost (intravenous prostaglandin)
   e Heparin

2.24 A 30-year-old lorry driver presents complaining of ulcers in the nail folds of his fourth and fifth fingers and pallor and tingling of his fingers when they are exposed to the cold. He smokes 35 cigarettes a day and is otherwise well. Examination reveals nicotine staining around his fingers and dry ulcers on the fourth and fifth digits; upper-limb pulses are all palpable. The most likely diagnosis is:
a Hyperhidrosis
b Thoracic outlet syndrome
c Buerger's disease
d Takayasu's arteritis
e Raynaud's disease

2.25 Which of the following disorders is more common in women than in men?
a Takayasu's arteritis
b Lymphoedema congenita
c Aortic dissection
d Hyperhidrosis
e Carotid body tumour

2.26 A 60-year-old Afro-Caribbean man is admitted to A&E complaining of a severe 'tearing' intrascapular pain, which came on suddenly. He has a medical history of hypertension, for which he takes bendrofluazide 2.5 mg once daily. On examination, his blood pressure is 170/90 mmHg from the right arm and 145/70 mmHg from the left arm, and his heart rate is 100 bpm. His ECG demonstrates no acute changes, and his chest X-ray reveals a widened mediastinum. The most likely diagnosis is:
a Rupture of the oesophagus
b Ruptured thoracic aortic aneurysm
c Mediastinitis
d Aortic dissection
e Cardiac tamponade

2.27 Which of the following statements is true regarding carotid artery disease?
   a A stenosis of 100% of the internal carotid artery warrants surgery.
   b Presence of a carotid bruit is a reliable indicator of stenosis.
   c Atherosclerotic lesions typically occur at the carotid bifurcation.
   d Damage to the hypoglossal nerve during carotid endarterectomy leads to weakness of the tongue on the contralateral side.
   e Stroke is not a recognised complication of surgery.

2.28 A 45-year-old truck driver is seen in clinic complaining of bilateral buttock and thigh claudication at 50 yards (46 metres). He confides that he has recently become impotent. He is a smoker and has a medical history of hypertension, for which he takes amlodipine 5 mg once daily. On examination, he has weak femoral and absent popliteal and pedal pulses. His feet are pale and cool. Duplex confirms your diagnosis. The most appropriate intervention would be:
   a Femoral-crural bypass
   b Axillo-unifem bypass
   c Bilateral femoral angioplasty
   d Femoral-popliteal bypass
   e Aorto-bifemoral bypass

2.29 Which of the following is an early feature of acute lower-limb ischaemia?
   a Fixed mottling
   b Pain on passive movement of the limb
   c Paralysis
   d Pallor
   e Paraesthesia

2.30 A 19-year-old is bought in by ambulance following an assault. He is confused, with a blood pressure of 70/40 mmHg and a heart rate of 120 bpm. On further examination, you notice he has a stab wound medial to his left nipple. In addition, his JVP is raised. The most appropriate next step is:
   a Urgent chest X-ray
   b Arterial blood gas
   c Insert a central line to more accurately assess JVP
   d Needle thoracocentesis
   e Pericardiocentesis

ANSWERS

2.1 The correct answer is A.

Varicose veins are dilated, tortuous veins of the superficial venous system. Sapheno-femoral incompetence is more common (seen in approximately 90%) than incompetence at the sapheno-popliteal junction in primary varicose veins. Damage to the saphenous nerve results in an area of sensory loss over the medial aspect of the calf, above the medial malleolus. Although deep vein thrombosis can cause varicose veins, it is not a *common* cause.

2.2 The correct answer is D.

Compartment syndrome due to reperfusion syndrome is a well-recognised complication following revascularisation (i.e. post-embolectomy) and is a surgical emergency. Symptoms are due to a raised intrafascial compartment pressure (>30 mmHg), which can lead to irreversible ischaemic necrosis of muscles and nerves crossing through the affected compartment. Clinical features include severe pain out of proportion to the injury; pain on passive stretch of the muscles within the compartment; and other signs of acute limb ischaemia. Four-compartment fasciotomy is the treatment of choice.

2.3 The correct answer is E.

Critical limb ischaemia is defined by the European Working Group on Critical Leg Ischaemia as the presence of ischaemic rest pain requiring analgesia for more than two weeks, or ulceration, or gangrene of the lower extremity where the absolute ankle systolic blood pressure is <50 mmHg and/or the toe systolic pressure is <30 mmHg (i.e. symptoms are due to objectively proven arterial occlusive disease).

2.4 The correct answer is C.

Intermittent claudication is reproducible ischaemic muscle pain that is classically bought on by walking and relieved by rest. It affects 5% of men over the age of 50 and is a common presentation of peripheral vascular disease. Treatment is medical, with intervention reserved for select cases e.g. patients with debilitating symptoms. Invasive imaging, i.e. angiography, should not be performed unless intervention is being considered.

2.5 The correct answer is D.

Further imaging is required prior to carotid endarterectomy. Carotid duplex is the preferred first-line imaging modality. CT scan of the brain is not useful in cases of transient ischaemic attack (TIA).

2.6 The correct answer is D.

The most likely diagnosis in an elderly, hypotensive male is a ruptured AAA. A profoundly hypotensive patient should not undergo CT scanning (which is often described as the 'doughnut of death') and is not fit for transfer to another hospital. FAST scanning, although able to assess for an aneurysm, cannot accurately detect rupture. Hypotensive resuscitation is often advocated in cases of ruptured AAAs.

2.7 The correct answer is A.

Reverse Trendelenburg is thought to reduce the risk of air embolus.

2.8 The correct answer is A.

Acute limb ischaemia may be caused by a thrombus or an embolus; management includes investigations geared towards establishing a cause. Urinalysis is useful for demonstrating myoglobinuria, since rhabdomyolysis is a well-recognised complication. Heparin should be administered intravenously.

2.9 The correct answer is D.

Approximately 80–5% of all leg ulcers in the UK are venous in aetiology.

2.10 The correct answer is C.

Operative mortality will be affected by the patient's co-morbidity. The operative mortality associated with elective AAA is between 1.2% and 8.4%.

2.11 The correct answer is C.

Ankle brachial pressure index should be assessed to exclude arterial disease. Venous ulcers typically occur in the gaitor region and overlie the medial malleolus. Venous duplex is indicated in patients with recurrent or complicated varicose veins, short saphenous incompetence or suspected deep venous insufficiency. The mainstay of management is leg elevation and compression bandaging. Skin grafting is performed in selected cases.

2.12 The correct answer is A.

This patient has a history suggestive of temporal arteritis (also known as giant cell arteritis) – a systemic vasculitis that primarily affects medium and large arteries. Features include new-onset headache, tenderness overlying the temporal artery, jaw claudication, an elevated ESR and, most devastatingly, visual loss. If temporal arteritis is suspected, treatment with high-dose steroids should be commenced in order to avoid visual loss. Definitive diagnosis is obtained by biopsy of the affected (usually temporal) artery, and this can be performed at a later stage.

2.13 The correct answer is C.

In view of the fact that the patient has an extensive femoral deep vein thrombosis, she is likely to have had a pulmonary embolus. It would be useful to establish whether she is therapeutic in terms of her warfarin, as it is likely that she is suboptimally anticoagulated.

2.14 The correct answer is D.

Physical signs of cardiac tamponade include neck vein distension, tachycardia, tachypnoea, pericardial rub, Beck's triad (i.e. increased jugular venous pressure, hypotension and diminished heart sounds), pulsus paradoxus, occasionally Kussmaul's sign and abolition of the y descent of the jugular venous or right atrial waveform. Note that not all of these will necessarily be present.

2.15 The correct answer is B.

A patient with an asymptomatic AAA does not require emergent referral to the vascular surgeons. An ultrasound scan of the abdominal aorta is the first-line screening investigation of choice and is used to monitor AAA growth.

2.16 The correct answer is B.

Other indications for AAA repair are growth rate >1.0 cm per year and the development of symptoms.

2.17 The correct answer is C.

Graded compression stockings, although not a cure for varicose veins, provide symptomatic relief. They reduce leg swelling and can prevent complications. A venous duplex is indicated in complex or recurrent venous disease. Venous ulceration and other secondary venous tissue changes, e.g. lipodermatosclerosis, are indications for surgical intervention.

2.18 The correct answer is E.

The patient has an acutely ischaemic leg – this is a surgical emergency. The most likely cause is an embolus, as the patient is in atrial fibrillation. Urgent referral to the vascular surgeons, intravenous heparin and embolectomy either with or without on-table angiography are required.

2.19 The correct answer is C.

The patient has symptoms, signs and risk factors supporting the diagnosis of a deep vein thrombosis (DVT). Therapeutic-dose heparin should be commenced on the clinical suspicion of a DVT. DVT should be subsequently confirmed with venous duplex imaging. There is no suggestion that the patient has had a pulmonary embolus, so CT pulmonary angiogram is not indicated. Heparin should be discontinued once therapeutic levels of warfarin are reached, and warfarin should be continued for six months.

2.20 The correct answer is A.

The greatest risk factor for aneurysm formation is thought to be smoking. AAAs are more common amongst Caucasians and are approximately five times more common in men than in women. Popliteal aneurysms are the most common peripheral artery aneurysm, affecting 10% of patients with an AAA. Popliteal aneurysms rarely rupture, and complications arise due to thrombosis or embolisation distally causing lower-limb ischaemia. Splenic artery aneurysms are more common in women.

2.21 The correct answer is C.

After wound swabs for culture, broad-spectrum antibiotics should be commenced in the first instance. Gram-positive cocci such as *Staphylococcus aureus*, group B *Streptococcus pyogenes*, group A *Streptococcus agalactiae* and methicillin-resistant *Staphylococcus aureus* (found in patients previously hospitalised) are the most commonly implicated organisms. If osteomyelitis is suspected, it may be useful to first X-ray the foot then perform an MRI. Amputation is indicated if there is spreading infection, failure of antibiotic therapy or gas gangrene. Dry, not wet, gangrene usually autoamputates.

2.22 The correct answer is A.

The nematode *Wuchereria bancrofti* is responsible for filariasis. Milroy's disease is a cause of primary lymphoedema, which is rare. The others are causes of secondary lymphoedema.

2.23 The correct answer is E.

The patient has Raynaud's disease. This is an idiopathic vasospastic condition that usually affects young women. When secondary to another condition, e.g. systemic lupus erythematosus or rheumatoid arthritis, it is termed Raynaud's syndrome.

2.24 The correct answer is C.

Buerger's disease (thromboangiitis obliterans) is an arterio-occlusive disease that affects the medium and small arteries of the upper and lower limbs. It typically affects young males and is clearly linked with smoking.

2.25 The correct answer is A.

Takayasu's arteritis is a chronic inflammatory disease that affects the aorta and its main branches; it is sometimes called 'pulseless arteritis'. It is more common in women and Asians.

2.26 The correct answer is D.

An aortic dissection is a tear in the intima that results in a connection between the aortic lumen and the media. Propagation of the dissection longitudinally and a re-entry tear result in the formation of a true lumen, lined by intima, and a false lumen, between the intima and media. Aortic dissections are more common in men, and predisposing factors include hypertension, connective-tissue disorders, pregnancy and trauma. They may be categorised according to their location using the DeBakey (types I, II and III) and Stanford (types A and B) classifications.

2.27 The correct answer is C.

The aim of surgery is to reduce the risk of stroke. An occluded carotid artery has no thromboembolic potential. Two-thirds of patients with a critical stenosis will not have a bruit. Damage to the hypoglossal nerve during carotid endarterectomy leads to weakness of the tongue on the same side. Stroke is an important complication of surgical intervention.

2.28 The correct answer is E.

The patient has symptoms suggestive of distal aorta and iliac (aortoiliac) occlusion, otherwise known as Leriche's syndrome. Leriche's syndrome is a classic triad of buttock/thigh claudication, impotence and absent/diminished femoral pulses.

2.29 The correct answer is D.

The others are late signs. Fixed mottling, muscle rigidity and pain on passive movement of the limb suggest irreversibility of the ischaemia. Pallor, pain and an objective temperature level are early signs of acute limb ischaemia.

2.30 The correct answer is E.

The patient has a history and signs suggestive of cardiac tamponade (accumulation of fluid in the pericardial space). The classic presentation of Beck's triad of hypotension, raised jugular venous pressure and muffled heart sounds, is typically seen in acute cardiac tamponade.

3

Urology

QUESTIONS

3.1 Which of the following statements is NOT true regarding poly-cystic kidneys?
  a The condition is characterised by multiple cysts in both kidneys.
  b There is a strong association with intracranial berry aneurysms.
  c Polycystic kidney disease usually presents between 30 and 60 years of age.
  d The condition is most commonly inherited as an autosomal-dominant form.
  e Ultrasonography is of no use in the diagnosis.

3.2 A 25-year-old man presents to A&E with a history of sudden-onset right-sided colicky loin-to-groin pain. What is the first investigation of choice?
  a Intravenous urography (IVU)
  b Plain abdominal X-ray
  c Urine dipstick
  d CT scan of the abdomen
  e Cystoscopy

3.3 What is the most common composition of urinary calculi?
  a Oxalate
  b Phosphate
  c Urate
  d Cystine
  e Carbonate

3.4   A 35-year-old man presents to his GP with symptoms of frequency and dysuria. Which of the following investigations is NOT appropriate?
a Urine microscopy and culture
b MRI scan of the renal tract
c Ultrasound scan of the renal tract
d Plain abdominal X-ray
e Cystoscopy

3.5   Malignant renal tumours in adults are most commonly:
a Nephroblastomas
b Adenocarcinomas
c Transitional cell tumours
d Squamous carcinomas
e Papillomas

3.6   Which of the following statements is true regarding abscesses of the renal cortex?
a Ascending infection is most often the cause.
b *E. coli* is the responsible organism in most cases.
c The kidney is never palpable.
d Urine is frequently sterile.
e Conservative management with intravenous antibiotics alone is indicated.

3.7   Which of the following statements is true regarding bladder diverticula?
a Most are congenital.
b Acquired bladder diverticula have all layers of the bladder wall.
c The majority of bladder diverticula are symptomatic.
d Cystoscopy can be used to diagnose bladder diverticula.
e 95% of bladder diverticula are found in women.

3.8   Ninety per cent of malignant bladder tumours in the developed world are:
a Squamous carcinomas
b Sarcomas
c Adenocarcinomas
d Transitional cell carcinomas
e Small-cell carcinomas

3.9 Which of the following is NOT a risk factor for malignant bladder cancers?
a Schistosomiasis
b Occupational exposure to aniline dye
c Cigarette smoking
d Alcohol
e Ectopia vesicae

3.10 Low-risk superficial bladder transitional cell carcinomas (TCCs) are first treated with:
a Intravesical BCG therapy
b Endoscopic resection
c Intravesical mitomycin
d Radiotherapy
e Cystectomy

3.11 Which of the following drugs is NOT an α-blocker?
a Finasteride
b Tamsulosin
c Doxazosin
d Indoramin
e Prazosin

3.12 Which of the following statements is true regarding prostate carcinoma?
a Prostate carcinoma is relatively uncommon in the elderly.
b Prostate carcinoma is always symptomatic.
c Prostate-specific antigen (PSA) is not useful as a tumour marker.
d Radical prostatectomy is the treatment of choice.
e Gonadotrophin-releasing hormone (GnRH) agonists are the mainstay of treatment in metastatic disease.

3.13 The organism most commonly responsible for bacterial prostatitis is:
a *Mycobacterium tuberculosii*
b *Staphylococcus aureus*
c Parvovirus
d *Escherichia coli*
e *Streptococcus pyogenes*

3.14 A 60-year-old man presents to urology outpatients with a several-month history of perineal pain, pain on ejaculation and urinary frequency. Urine samples have not cultured any organisms, so the likely diagnosis is:
   a Acute bacterial prostatitis
   b Chronic pelvic pain syndrome
   c Benign prostatic hypertrophy
   d Chronic bacterial prostatitis
   e Bladder neck obstruction

3.15 A 20-year-old man presents to his GP with a four-hour history of sudden-onset, severe right-sided testicular pain. On examination, the affected testis is swollen, painful to touch and lying high in the scrotum. What should the GP do?
   a Reassure the patient and send him home with analgesia.
   b Prescribe antibiotics for the treatment of acute epididymitis and send him home.
   c Organise an urgent Doppler ultrasound scan of the scrotum at the nearest hospital.
   d Refer immediately to the surgeon on-call for scrotal exploration at the nearest hospital.

3.16 Which of the following statements is true of testicular seminomas?
   a Seminomas arise from primitive totipotent germ cells.
   b Seminomas usually present after 60 years of age.
   c Macroscopically, the tumour appears cystic.
   d Seminomas are highly radiosensitive.
   e Seminomas usually metastasise to the brain.

3.17 Which of the following statements is NOT true regarding testicular teratomas?
   a Teratomas tend to affect a younger age group, peak incidence being 20–30 years of age.
   b Teratomas can present as hydrocoeles.
   c Teratomas rarely spread to the lung and the liver.
   d Teratomas usually produce α-fetoprotein.
   e Following orchidectomy, teratomas are treated by combination chemotherapy.

3.18 Which of the following is a possible complication of testicular maldescent?
a Increased risk of torsion
b Increased risk of trauma
c Increased risk of malignant disease
d Inguinal hernia
e All of the above

3.19 Which of the following statements is true regarding varicocoeles?
a There is a higher incidence in infertile men.
b Varicocoeles are present in up to 50% of men.
c Varicocoeles are always asymptomatic.
d Varicocoeles usually occur on the right.
e Varicocoeles always require treatment.

3.20 The commonest blood-borne agent to infect the testis is:
a Cytomegalovirus
b Mumps virus
c Herpes simplex virus
d Epstein-Barr virus
e Herpes zoster virus

3.21 The most common presentation of bladder cancer is with:
a Painful haematuria
b Frequency
c Painless haematuria
d Recurrent cystitis
e Urgency

3.22 Which of the following statements is true regarding torsion of the testes?
a The testicle is likely to be salvageable if duration of the torsion is 12 hours.
b Pain and absence of the cremasteric reflex support the diagnosis.
c Urinary symptoms are common.
d It more commonly occurs on the right.
e Peak incidence is in infancy.

3.23 A 66-year-old man presents to his GP complaining of discomfort in the left loin and of frank haematuria. On examination, he is pale, blood pressure is 200/110 mmHg and heart rate is 70 bpm. Abdominal examination reveals a left varicocoele. The most likely diagnosis is:
a Pyelonephritis
b Wilms' tumour
c Renal colic
d Renal cell carcinoma (RCC)
e Von Hippel-Lindau disease

3.24 A 35-year-old male motorcyclist is involved in a road traffic accident. He has sustained a fracture to his pelvis. Features suggestive of a urethral injury do NOT include:
a High-riding prostate on digital rectal examination
b Presence of blood at the urethral meatus
c Perineal bruising
d Frank haematuria
e Suprapubic tenderness

3.25 A 70-year-old man is immediately post-op transurethral resection of prostate (TURP). You are called to review him, as he has suddenly become confused and is vomiting. He complains of nausea and seeing 'flashing lights'. On examination, he is apyrexial, blood pressure is 120/70 mmHg and heart rate is 60 bpm. The most likely diagnosis is:
a TUR syndrome
b Urinary tract infection
c Sepsis
d Halothane-induced hepatotoxicity
e Opiate-induced confusion

3.26 A 75-year-old man presents to A&E with a one-day history of increasing lower abdominal pain and inability to pass urine. He reports that prior to the episode, his urinary stream has been poor and he often has to strain to completely empty his bladder. On examination, he is in extreme discomfort, blood pressure is 140/70 mmHg and heart rate is 110 bpm. He is markedly tender suprapubically, and the bladder is palpable at the umbilicus. The most appropriate next step is:

a Bladder ultrasound scan
b Intramuscular morphine for pain
c Urine dipstick
d PSA
e Urinary catheterisation

ANSWERS

3.1 The correct answer is E.

Ultrasonography is very accurate in detecting multiple cysts in adults.

3.2 The correct answer is C.

The patient most likely has renal colic. A urine dipstick test is necessary to confirm the presence of haematuria, which is almost always present in renal colic. If haematuria is present, a plain abdominal X-ray (note that 10% of renal stones are not visualised on plain X-ray) followed by an IVU can be arranged. Alternatively, a CT scan of the kidneys, ureters and bladder can be performed.

3.3 The correct answer is A.

Approximately 60% of stones are oxalate, 33% are phosphate, 5% are urate and 1% are cystine.

3.4 The correct answer is B.

The patient has symptoms suggestive of a urinary tract infection. Urine cultures are necessary to identify the causative organism, which is usually bowel flora. Ultrasound scan of the bladder and kidneys may reveal dilatation of the upper tracts. A plain abdominal X-ray can help to identify bladder stones, and cystoscopy can reveal bladder diverticula.

3.5 The correct answer is B.

3.6 The correct answer is D.

Carbuncles of the kidney represent haematogenous infection, usually *Staphylococcus aureus*, coming from a primary focus such as a cutaneous boil. There is usually toxaemia, pyrexia and loin tenderness, and the kidney may be palpable. Percutaneous drainage and antibiotics are indicated once the diagnosis is made.

3.7 The correct answer is D.

Most bladder diverticula are found in men and are acquired rather then congenital. Only congenital bladder diverticula possess all layers of the bladder wall rather than just the mucosa. Most are clinically silent.

3.8 The correct answer is D.

In the developing world, 75% of bladder cancers are squamous cell carcinomas.

3.9 The correct answer is D.

3.10 The correct answer is B.

For bladder TCC that does not invade the bladder wall or that only invades the lamina propria (pTa or pT1 tumours), endoscopic resection is carried out initially, followed by intravesical mitomycin therapy to prevent recurrence.

3.11 The correct answer is A.

Finasteride is a 5-α-reductase inhibitor that blocks the conversion of testosterone to its active metabolite in the prostate. It leads to a reduction in prostate size and thereby improves urinary flow rates. It can take up to six months to show beneficial effects.

3.12 The correct answer is E.

Prostate carcinoma is relatively *common* in the elderly, and it can be completely asymptomatic. PSA is a useful tumour marker, particularly when tracking the patient's response to treatment. Radical prostatectomy is generally reserved for young patients with a high chance of localised disease.

3.13 The correct answer is D.

3.14 The correct answer is B.

3.15 The correct answer is D.

The presumptive diagnosis is that of testicular torsion, and consequently it is best to explore the scrotum as soon as possible. If the testis is viable, it is untwisted and sutured to the tunica vaginalis. If it is infarcted, it is removed.

3.16 The correct answer is D.

Seminomas arise from cells of the seminiferous tubules and usually present between 30 and 40 years of age. Macroscopically, the tumour is solid and looks like a cut potato on section.

3.17 The correct answer is C.

Teratomas spread relatively early to the lungs and liver.

3.18 The correct answer is E.

These are all possible complications of maldescent.

3.19 The correct answer is A.

Varicocoeles are present in up to 10% of men, usually occur on the right and can cause a dragging sensation in the scrotum. They do not usually require treatment but can be cured radiologically by embolising the testicular vein or surgically by ligating and dividing all testicular veins.

3.20 The correct answer is B.

3.21 The correct answer is C.

Bladder cancer typically presents with painless macroscopic haematuria. Irritative symptoms of urgency, frequency and dysuria may also be present. Pelvic or bony pain is seen in advanced disease.

3.22 The correct answer is B.

Salvage of the testicle is most likely if duration of the torsion is <6–8 hours. The most common presentation seen in A&E is that of acute-onset pain, which may be associated with nausea and vomiting. Urinary symptoms are uncommon. In adolescents, the left testis is more commonly affected. Peak incidence is in adolescence.

3.23 The correct answer is D.

Renal cell carcinoma (RCC) (also known as clear cell carcinoma or Gravitz's tumour) is an adenocarcinoma. Peak incidence is in the sixth to eighth decade. The classic triad of symptoms in RCC is haematuria, loin pain and a palpable abdominal mass – and these suggest advanced disease. RCC is, however, usually asymptomatic. Other symptoms include: weight loss; anaemia (due to haematuria); varicocoele (due to obstruction of the testicular vein by tumour invading the left renal vein); and paraneoplastic syndromes, e.g. hypertension (due to renin secretion by the tumour), hypercalcaemia (due to ectopic PTH-like substance secretion) and polycythaemia (due to ectopic erythropoietin secretion). Wilms' tumours have a similar presentation but occur in childhood. Von Hippel-Lindau syndrome is a risk factor for the development of RCC.

3.24 The correct answer is E.

Retrograde urethrography is useful for assessing the extent of urethral injury.

3.25 The correct answer is A.

TUR syndrome complicates approximately 0.5% of cases of TURP, and it occurs because of excessive absorption of the hypotonic irrigation fluid used during the procedure. This results in a dilutional hyponatraemia and the subsequent symptoms.

3.26 The correct answer is E.

The patient is in acute urinary retention. Given his history, this is most likely secondary to bladder outflow obstruction, e.g. benign prostatic hyperplasia or prostate cancer. Immediate management to relieve his symptoms is urethral catherisation. Should this fail, suprapubic catheterisation should be performed; the residual volume must be recorded, and this will help give the diagnosis. Urinalysis (for infection), rectal examination (for assessment of the prostate), PSA and renal tract ultrasound (for hydronephrosis) may be performed subsequently to establish a cause.

Breast and Endocrine Surgery

QUESTIONS

4.1 The following features of breast cancer suggest a poor prognosis, EXCEPT:
a Negative oestrogen receptor status
b Positive human epidermal growth factor receptor (HER-2) status
c Bloody nipple discharge
d Large tumour size
e Axillary lymph node metastasis

4.2 A 22-year-old woman presents to clinic with a one-month history of a lump in her right breast. Examination reveals a mobile, firm, smooth and non-tender lump of 2 cm in the lower outer quadrant. No axillary lymph nodes are palpable, and she has no risk factors or family history of breast cancer. The most likely diagnosis is:
a Fibroadenoma
b Lobular breast cancer
c Fibroadenosis with a breast cyst
d Duct ectasia
e Phyllodes tumour

4.3 Which of the following is true regarding the UK breast-screening programme?
a All women aged between 55 to 69 years are invited.
b Breast screening only detects non-treatable breast cancer.
c Breast screening is performed two-yearly.
d Breast screening does not improve overall mortality, but it does improve morbidity.
e Two-view mammography is performed.

4.4 The organism most commonly implicated in mastitis is:

a *Escherichia coli*

b *Staphylococcus aureus*

c *Streptococcus pyogenes*

d *Pseudomonas aeruginosa*

e *Candida albicans*

4.5 Which of the following is associated with an increased risk of developing breast cancer?

a Increasing age

b Obesity

c Early menarche

d Alcohol excess

e All of the above

4.6 A 36-year-old woman presents to A&E with a two-day history of a tender lump in the left breast, and today she has been feverish. Examination confirms the presence of a lump that is 3 cm by 5 cm, warm, well circumscribed and tender. There is associated skin erythema. The most appropriate next step is:

a Mammography

b Ultrasound-guided or clinical aspiration of the lump

c Incision and drainage of the presumed abscess

d Commence antibiotics and observe

e Await microbiology cultures and commence the appropriate antibiotics

4.7 A 50-year-old woman is seen in clinic complaining of a three-week history of spontaneous discharge of serosanguinous fluid from the left nipple. She has no risk factors or family history of breast cancer. On examination, a bloodstained discharge can be expressed from a single duct in the left nipple. No discrete lumps or axillary lymph nodes are palpable. Which of the following is not appropriate in the immediate management of the patient?

a Reassure and discharge

b Microdochectomy

c Send nipple discharge for urgent microscopy and culture

d Ultrasound scan of the left breast

e Mammography

4.8 A 66-year-old woman presents with a well-circumscribed, painless lump in the upper outer quadrant of her left breast. Her last mammogram was performed a year ago and was entirely normal. Which of the following statements is true?
   a Repeat mammography is not required, since the last one was performed only a year ago.
   b Ultrasound is not useful, given her age.
   c Fixity of the lump to underlying structures suggests it is likely to be malignant.
   d Phyllodes tumour is the most likely diagnosis.
   e Blood tests for tumour markers should be sent.

4.9 A 49-year-old is two weeks post-op right mastectomy and axillary clearance for breast cancer. She presents in clinic complaining of difficulty with particular movements. On examination, she has winging of the right scapula. The most likely cause of her symptoms is damage to the:
   a Median nerve
   b Axillary nerve
   c Long thoracic nerve
   d Thoracodorsal nerve
   e Intercostobrachial nerve

4.10 The most common site of metastases of breast cancer is the:
   a Brain
   b Liver
   c Lung
   d Bone
   e Stomach

4.11 A 67-year-old woman is five days post-op excision of a left breast lump and axillary clearance. She is seen in clinic complaining of a swelling in the left axilla and is concerned that the cancer has recurred. On examination, there is fullness in the left axilla that extends into the mastectomy wound. The most appropriate next step is:
   a Ultrasound scan of the swelling
   b Aspiration of the swelling
   c Prescribe antibiotics
   d Mammography
   e Physiotherapy

4.12 A 30-year-old woman has recently undergone genetic screening and has been found to be BRCA1 positive. The following advice should be given regarding breast cancer surveillance:
  a She requires yearly mammograms only from age 30 to 49 years.
  b She requires three-yearly mammograms only from age 30 to 49 years.
  c She requires yearly ultrasound and mammography from age 30 to 49 years.
  d She requires three-yearly MRI and mammography from age 30 to 49 years.
  e She requires yearly MRI and mammography from age 30 to 49 years.

4.13 A 41-year-old woman presents in clinic with a four-month history of bilateral breast pain and tenderness that is worse before her periods and keeps her awake at night. She has no risk factors or family history of breast cancer. On examination, both breasts are diffusely tender, and no discrete lumps are palpable within either the breasts or axillae. Which of the following drugs would NOT be useful in her management?
  a Danazol
  b Non-steroidal anti-inflammatory drugs
  c Prednisolone
  d Bromocriptine
  e Tamoxifen

4.14 A 69-year-old man is seen in clinic with a six-month history of swelling of the right breast. He is otherwise fit and well. On examination, the right breast is diffusely enlarged and no discrete lump is palpable within either the breast or axilla. Examination of the external genitalia is unremarkable. An ultrasound scan confirms right-sided gynaecomastia. The most appropriate next step is:
  a Observe
  b Mammography
  c Reduction mammoplasty
  d Bloods tests for sex hormones
  e Commence tamoxifen

4.15 Which of the following statements is true regarding breast cancer in men?
  a It has an equal incidence to breast cancer in women.
  b It is associated with kidney disease.
  c Men with Klinefelter's syndrome are at higher risk.
  d Sarcomas are the most common tumour type.
  e It tends to be diagnosed at an earlier stage in men than in women.

4.16 A 50-year-old woman is three days post-op total thyroidectomy for follicular carcinoma of the thyroid gland and is admitted confused and complaining of tingling in her fingertips and perioral region, cramps in her calves and lethargy. On examination, the surgical scar is intact and clean, her blood pressure is 120/70 mmHg and her heart rate is 70 bpm. The most useful investigation is:
  a Chest X-ray
  b Blood test for parathyroid hormone
  c Blood tests for thyroid function
  d Ultrasound of the wound
  e Blood test for serum calcium

4.17 A 56-year-old woman with a history of locally invasive breast cancer is admitted with confusion, polydipsia, urinary frequency, constipation and back pain. The most likely diagnosis is:
  a Hepatic encephalopathy secondary to metastases
  b Acute renal failure
  c Cerebral metastases
  d Hypercalcaemia
  e Hypoglycaemia

4.18 The classic feature seen in hypercalcaemia is:
  a ST depression
  b Prolonged QT interval
  c $S_1 Q_3 T_3$
  d Shortened QT interval
  e Tented T waves

4.19 The following features increase the likelihood of a thyroid nodule being malignant, EXCEPT:
a History of radiation to the head and neck
b Male gender
c New-onset dysphagia
d Cervical lymphadenopathy
e Family history of MEN type 1 syndrome

4.20 Which of the following statements is true regarding thyroid cancer?
a An elevated serum calcitonin is suggestive of papillary carcinoma.
b Medullary thyroid cancer is the most common thyroid malignancy.
c A higher incidence of follicular cancer is seen in regions of low dietary iodine intake.
d Anaplastic tumours are typically slow-growing.
e Pain is often a feature.

4.21 A 25-year-old woman presents to her GP complaining of a three-month history of palpitations, weight loss, intolerance to heat and irritability. She has also noticed a lump in her neck. On examination, she is tachycardic and the thyroid gland is diffusely enlarged and non-tender; a bruit is audible over it. She has a medical history of pernicious anaemia but is otherwise well. Blood tests demonstrate elevated triiodothyronine (T3) and thyroxine (T4) and low TSH; antibodies for thyroid peroxidase are positive. The most likely diagnosis is:
a Graves' thyrotoxicosis
b Hashimoto's thyroiditis
c Toxic multinodular goitre
d Papillary thyroid cancer
e Lymphoma

4.22 A 40-year-old Caucasian woman from Derbyshire complains to her GP of some difficulty swallowing; her partner has also noticed that her neck is swollen. She is otherwise fit and well. On examination, she is clinically euthyroid and the thyroid gland is diffusely enlarged and non-tender. Blood tests demonstrate normal TSH, T3 and T4; and antibodies for thyroid peroxidase are negative. The most likely diagnosis is:

a Riedel's thyroiditis
b Lymphoma
c Plummer's disease
d Hashimoto's thyroiditis
e Simple colloid goitre

4.23 Which of the following statements is true regarding phaechromocytomas?

a They are a common cause of hypertension.
b 3% are bilateral.
c They arise from the adrenal cortex.
d They may occur in association with von Hippel-Lindau disease.
e 50% are extra-adrenal.

4.24 In primary hyperparathyroidism, the expected biochemical abnormality is:

	Serum calcium	Serum PTH	Serum phosphate	Serum chloride
a	High	High	Low	High
b	High	High	High	High
c	Low	High	Low	High
d	High	High	Low	Low
e	High	High	High	Low

4.25 Which of the following statements is true regarding multiple endocrine neoplasia syndrome (MEN)?

a MEN type 1 is due to a chromosomal abnormality located on chromosome 13.
b Hyperparathyroidism occurs more commonly in MEN type 2A than in MEN type 1.
c MEN is more common in women.
d The pattern of inheritance depends on the type.
e Medullary thyroid cancer is associated with MEN type 2.

4.26 The least common site of presentation of breast cancer is the:
  a Upper outer quadrant
  b Subareolar region
  c Upper inner quadrant
  d Lower outer quadrant
  e Lower inner quadrant

4.27 A 76-year-old woman presents in clinic with a three-month history of a palpable lump in her thyroid gland. She denies any symptoms of dysphagia or dysphonia or any symptoms suggestive of hypo- or hyperthyroidism. On examination, there is a 1 cm nodule within the left lobe of the thyroid gland and she is clinically euthyroid. The most appropriate next step is:
  a Reassure
  b Ultrasound and FNA cytology
  c Thyroid scintigraphy
  d Excision biopsy
  e CT scan for retrosternal extension

4.28 A patient is referred to clinic with suspected acromegaly. Which of the following tests would NOT aid your diagnosis?
  a Growth-hormone level
  b Insulin-like growth-factor 1 (IGF-1) level
  c Spinal X-ray
  d Pituitary MRI
  e HbA1c

4.29 A young woman presents to clinic with a history of headaches, acne, increased facial hair growth, weight gain and cessation of menses. On examination, she has a round, full face and purple marks on her abdomen and breasts. The most likely clinical diagnosis is:
  a Conn's disease
  b Acromegaly
  c Thyrotoxicosis
  d Cushing's disease
  e Hypothyroid

4.30 Which of the following is NOT a manifestation of a pituitary adenoma?
   a Bitemporal hemianopia
   b Cushing's disease
   c Hypergonadism
   d Impotence
   e Acromegaly

4.31 Which of the following findings would NOT support the diagnosis of Addisonian crisis?
   a Neutropoenia
   b Hypoglycaemia
   c Hyponatraemia
   d Hyperkalaemia
   e Metabolic acidosis

4.32 Which of the following is NOT a common cause of primary hypogonadism?
   a Klinefelter's syndrome
   b Kallmann's syndrome
   c Undescended testes
   d Mumps orchitis
   e Haemochromatosis

4.33 A 63-year-old woman presents with a history of constipation, episodes of confusion, polydipsia and polyuria. Blood tests reveal an elevated plasma calcium level. She has a medical history of renal calculi. The most likely diagnosis is:
   a Type 2 diabetes mellitus
   b Diabetes insipidus
   c Hyperparathyroidism
   d Conn's syndrome
   e Thyrotoxicosis

ANSWERS

4.1   The correct answer is C.

The Nottingham Prognostic Index is a useful prognostic indicator in breast cancer, and it takes into account tumour size, spread (i.e. stage) and histological grade. Oestrogen and progesterone receptor positivity and HER-2 negativity are associated with better outcomes and are useful for guiding treatment.

4.2   The correct answer is A.

Fibroadenomas classically occur in the 15–25 age group. They are typically firm, rubbery, painless and well circumscribed, and they are usually 2–3 cm in diameter. Diagnosis for all breast lumps is by triple assessment – clinical examination, imaging (ultrasound in this case) and histology. Excision biopsy is indicated if age is >30 years, if the lump is increasing in size or at the patient's request.

4.3   The correct answer is E.

Breast screening detects early breast cancer. All women aged 50–70 are invited to attend breast screening every three years. A 35% reduction in mortality is seen in screened compared to unscreened patients aged between 50 and 70 years. Two-view mammography is thought to improve cancer detection rates by 43% compared to single-view mammography. The intention of the NHS Breast Screening Programme is to eventually screen all women aged 47–73 years old.

4.4   The correct answer is B.

Mastitis is commonly associated with breastfeeding. The underlying aetiology is milk stasis, and this can be complicated with infection. *Staphylococcus aureus* and *Staphylococcus albus* are the most commonly implicated organisms. Clinical features include breast pain, erythema and swelling with/without fever; a breast abscess may also be present.

4.5   The correct answer is E.

Age is the greatest risk factor for breast cancer after gender. Age (older) at first birth, nulliparity, late menopause, failure to breastfeed, current or recent HRT or OCP use, exposure to ionising radiation, higher socio-economic status and a personal or family history of breast cancer are all associated with an increased risk of breast cancer.

4.6   The correct answer is B.

The patient has a history and signs suggestive of a breast abscess. Drainage of the abscess, clinically or with ultrasound guidance, should be attempted, and multiple aspirations may be required for complete resolution of the abscess. Following aspiration, empirical antibiotics should be commenced pending culture and sensitivity results. Incision and drainage under a general anaesthetic should be performed if the overlying skin is not viable or if aspiration fails.

4.7   The correct answer is A.

Nipple discharge can be physiological or can represent ductal pathology. Serosanguinous discharge should raise concerns regarding breast cancer, and this risk increases with age. Other causes include duct ectasia and duct papilloma. All patients ≥35 years old should have mammography. Nipple-discharge cytology (rarely) and ultrasound of the retroareolar area may also be useful. Clinical examination should include confirmation of blood in the nipple discharge by cytology. Microdochectomy (excision of a single duct) or total duct excision (in older patients) should be considered following investigations.

4.8   The correct answer is E.

A breast lump should be assessed using triple assessment – clinical examination, imaging (mammogram and ultrasound) and biopsy to give cytology/histology. Breast cancer is the most important differential diagnosis in older patients. Nipple inversion, dimpling/tethering of the skin, bloody nipple discharge, ulceration, eczema, oedema (peau d'orange), hardness and fixity of the lump, and axillary lymphadenopathy raise the suspicion of breast cancer.

4.9   The correct answer is C.

Damage to the intercostobrachial nerves causes sensation loss in the skin overlying the medial aspect of the arm. Damage to the thoracodorsal nerve leads to weakness of the latissimus dorsi muscle. Damage to the long thoracic nerve of Bell, which innervates the serratus anterior muscle, leads to winging of the scapula.

4.10 The correct answer is D.

Bone is the most common site of metastases, followed by the lung and the liver.

4.11 The correct answer is B.

The patient has symptoms and signs suggestive of a seroma. This is a common post-op complication. Seromas may resolve either spontaneously or with serial aspiration.

4.12 The correct answer is E.

In patients with proven BRCA1 and BRCA2 mutations, annual MRI and mammography is recommended from age 30 to 49 years. In patients with proven TP53 mutation, annual MRI and mammography is recommended form age 20 to 49 years.

4.13 The correct answer is C.

The patient has cyclical mastalgia. Mastalgia is common and usually benign. Causes include premenstrual syndrome, fibrocystic disease, musculoskeletal pain (Tietze's syndrome) and, less commonly, cancer. Ultrasound and biopsy are indicated if pain is localised or if a lump is palpable; otherwise, management involves reassurance, as well as advice regarding support bras, diet and smoking cessation.

4.14 The correct answer is D.

Blood tests should be performed for liver function, thyroid function, oestrogen, testosterone, sex-hormone-binding globulin (SHBG), luteinising hormone (LH), follicle-stimulating hormone (FSH), prolactin and β-hCG in an attempt to establish the cause.

4.15 The correct answer is C.

Breast cancer in men is rare. Male breast cancer is associated with states in which there are lower androgen and higher oestrogen levels, such as liver cirrhosis and Klinefelter's syndrome (XXY). Male breast cancers tend to be diagnosed at a later stage than breast cancers in women, although prognosis is similar for tumours of the same stage.

4.16 The correct answer is E.

Hypocalcaemia secondary to hypoparathyroidism may occur as a result of either inadvertent removal of the parathyroid glands or compromise of the glands' blood supply. This is a complication of total thyroidectomy and typically occurs at day 3–5 post-operatively. Symptoms include carpopedal spasm, periorbital paraesthesia, confusion, irritability and seizures, amongst others. Chvostek's and Trousseau's signs may also be positive. ECG can demonstrate a prolonged QT interval and ST changes. The most useful first test is serum calcium, as this will guide management.

4.17 The correct answer is D.

The patient has symptoms of hypercalcaemia, which is likely to be secondary to bony metastases from a breast primary. Treatment options include rehydration, loop diuretics (e.g. furosemide) and bisphophonates (e.g. pamidronate).

4.18 The correct answer is D.

In hypercalcaemia, there is a shortened QT interval. In hypocalcaemia, the QT interval is prolonged. Tented T waves, a shortened QT interval and ST-segment depression are early features of hyperkalaemia. In hypokalaemia, the QRS complex is widened, there is ST depression and T wave flattening and large U waves. $S_1 Q_3 T_3$ is seen in pulmonary embolus.

4.19 The correct answer is E.

MEN types 2A and 2B are associated with medullary thyroid cancer. Other features suggestive of malignancy include a family history of medullary thyroid cancer (familial MTC); age <20 years or >70 years; rapid growth; associated dysphonia or cough; and fixity, hardness or an ill-defined nodule on palpation.

4.20 The correct answer is C.

Papillary carcinoma is the most common thyroid malignancy (accounting for approximately 80%), followed in order of incidence by follicular, medullary and anaplastic thyroid cancer. An elevated serum calcitonin is highly suggestive of medullary carcinoma, since unlike other thyroid cancers, medullary carcinoma is derived from the calcitonin-producing C cells of the thyroid. Anaplastic tumours are the most aggressive of all the thyroid cancers and are rapidly growing, often presenting with symptoms of local invasion, e.g. hoarseness of voice and dysphagia; prognosis is poor. Pain is more a feature of benign thyroid disease.

4.21 The correct answer is A.

The patient has features of hyperthyroidism. Graves' disease is the most common cause of thyrotoxicosis (accounting for approximately 70–80%); it is an autoimmune condition that typically presents in younger patients with a painless diffuse goitre and eye signs (e.g.

chemosis, proptosis, periorbital oedema, ophthalmoplegia, corneal ulceration). Other extrathyroidal manifestations include pretibial myxoedema and thyroid acropachy. In addition, approximately 50% have a family history of autoimmune disease. In Graves' disease, thyrotrophin receptor autoantibodies (TRAb) are produced and these bind to and activate the TSH receptor, leading to excess thyroxine secretion and thyrocyte proliferation. Antibodies for thyroid peroxidase are positive in autoimmune thyroid disease. Treatment includes β-blockers (for tachycardia), antithyroid medication (e.g. carbimazole), radioactive iodine and surgery in selected cases. Hashimoto's thyroiditis is an autoimmune disease that results in hypothyroidism. Cancers rarely present with hyperthyroidism.

4.22 The correct answer is E.

The patient has a simple colloid/endemic goitre. A goitre is a diffuse or nodular enlargement of the thyroid gland. Symptoms may be due to compression, e.g. dysphagia, stridor, neck vein distension, dizziness on arm elevation (Pemberton's sign), or to endocrine abnormalities, i.e. hypo- or hyperthyroidism. Goitres can be classified as sporadic or endemic and as toxic or non-toxic. The most common cause of endemic goitre is iodine deficiency and the presence of environmental or dietary goitrogens, e.g. vegetables of the *Brassica* family, such as cabbage. In England, endemic areas include the Chilterns, the Cotswolds, Derbyshire and Yorkshire, where iodide content of water and food has been historically low. Sporadic non-toxic goitres are typically asymptomatic; their cause is usually unknown but can include thyroiditis (e.g. post-partum, Riedel's, Hashimoto's), dyshormogenesis, drugs (i.e. goitrogens such as lithium), thyroid hormone resistance syndrome, genetic disorders (e.g. TSH receptor mutation), infiltration of the thyroid gland (e.g. sarcoidosis, amyloidosis) and malignancy.

4.23 The correct answer is D.

Phaechromocytomas are catecholamine-secreting tumours that arise from the chromaffin cells of the adrenal medulla. They are uncommon and are often described as the 10% tumour – as 10% are multiple, 10% are bilateral and 10% are familial. However, this view is outdated, as approximately 25% are bilateral. Phaechromocytomas can occur in association with MEN type 2 (MEN 2A and 2B), neurofibromatosis type 1 (von Recklinghausen's disease) and von Hippel-Lindau disease, all of which are autosomal-dominant disorders. Ninety per cent of phaechromocytomas are located within the adrenals and approximately 98% are intra-abdominal.

4.24 The correct answer is A.

Bone alkaline phosphatase and 24-hour urinary calcium excretion are also often elevated.

4.25 The correct answer is E.

The MENIN gene responsible for MEN type 1 is located on chromosome 11. Hyperparathyroidism is the most common presentation of MEN type 1, and it occurs due to hyperplasia of all four parathyroid glands. MEN is twice as common in men. Inheritance is autosomal dominant in MEN syndromes types 1 and 2.

4.26 The correct answer is E.

The least-common site of presentation of breast cancer is the lower inner quadrant. Breast cancers occur most frequently in the upper outer quadrant of the breast.

4.27 The correct answer is B.

Approximately 5–10% of solitary thyroid nodules are malignant, independent of size. Fine-needle aspiration biopsy should be performed when evaluating any thyroid nodule, with or without ultrasound guidance (more commonly the latter). In addition, a thyroid function test should be performed. Thyroid scintigraphy allows for the detection of areas of autonomously functioning thyroid tissue, and based on radionuclide uptake, nodules are classified as hyperfunctioning ('hot') or hypofunctioning ('cold'). 'Hot' nodules are almost never malignant, and only a small proportion of 'cold' nodules are malignant; thus the use of thyroid scintigraphy in diagnosing thyroid nodules is limited. CT scan may be useful for assessing retrosternal extension and absolute size in selected cases. Incisional biopsy should be avoided because of the potential risk of seeding and local recurrence.

4.28 The correct answer is E.

Growth hormone and IGF-1 levels would be elevated in acromegaly. A spinal radiograph may show abnormal bone growth. A pituitary MRI may show a benign tumour. While fasting glucose and glucose tolerance tests may prove abnormal, HbA1c will not necessarily be altered.

4.29 The correct answer is D.

Cushing's disease specifically refers to an ACTH-secreting pituitary adenoma resulting in elevated plasma levels of cortisol. This can manifest as weight gain; swelling of fat pads, often leading to a 'buffalo hump'; a round 'moon' face; thinning of the skin; purple or red striae; hirsutism; amenorrhoea; infertility; impotence; and reduced libido.

4.30 The correct answer is C.

Pressure on the optic chiasm classically produces a bitemporal hemianopia. Corticotrophic adenomas secrete adrenocorticotrophic hormone (ACTH), leading to Cushing's syndrome. Somatotrophic adenomas secrete growth hormone (GH), which can cause acromegaly, and prolactinomas can lead to impotence.

4.31 The correct answer is A.

Eosinophilia and lymphocytosis, NOT neutropoenia, are observed during an Addisonian crisis. The diminished aldosterone production causes the other results seen. The low aldosterone level leads to sodium loss and hydrogen ion reabsorption at the renal distal tubules.

4.32 The correct answer is B.

Klinefelter's syndrome is a genetic abnormality where two or more X chromosomes are present in a male. This leads to, amongst other things, underproduction of testosterone. In Kallmann's syndrome, there is abnormal development of the hypothalamus, and this is a cause of secondary hypogonadism. Both undescended testes and mumps may cause testicular damage, leading to dysfunction in later life. Haemochromatosis can cause testicular failure or pituitary gland dysfunction, leading to deranged testosterone levels.

4.33 The correct answer is C.

While all of the options may cause polydipsia and polyuria, only hyperparathyroidism causes the elevated calcium levels that explain all of the symptoms described.

5

Orthopaedics and Trauma, including Neurosurgery

QUESTIONS

5.1 A 30-year-old man is brought into the emergency department following a fight in which he was stabbed in the right side of his chest. He appears distressed and is very short of breath. On examination, he has a heart rate of 130 bpm, blood pressure is 80/60 mmHg, saturations are 95% on 15 L/min of oxygen with a respiratory rate of 30, and he has a raised JVP and prominent neck veins. His trachea is deviated to the left. On percussion, the right side of his chest is hyper-resonant, with no breath sounds on auscultation. The most appropriate course of action would be:

a Chest X-ray
b Arterial blood gas
c Insertion of a large-bore cannula in the right side of the chest
d Insertion of a large-bore cannula in the right/left arm
e Examination of the abdomen

5.2 A 50-year-old builder is working on a building site when he is struck on his arm by a falling piece of masonry. He attends the emergency department complaining of a painful arm, and there is some deformity. X-ray shows a fracture in the mid-shaft of the humerus. When examining him, you should pay particular attention to:

a Examining the power of the wrist flexors
b Examining the power of the wrist extensors
c Examining the sensation of the palm
d Examining the power of the shoulder abductors
e Examining the sensation of the little finger

5.3 A 52-year-old woman who had a right mastectomy for breast cancer four years ago is admitted with an acute episode of lower-back pain and is unable to mobilise. On examination, she is found to have reduced power in ankle dorsiflexion and planterflexion, absent ankle reflexes and altered perianal sensation. She is also found to be in urinary retention. The most appropriate investigation is:
a X-ray of the lumbosacral spine
b Nuclear medicine bone scan
c CT scan chest/abdomen/pelvis
d MRI of the spine
e Mammogram and ultrasound of the left breast

5.4 A 30-year-old woman who has fallen from her horse is brought into the emergency department by ambulance with a deformed right ankle. The X-ray shows a complex fracture-dislocation of the ankle. When you examine her, you notice the right foot is pale, with a capillary refill time of greater than five seconds, and she has altered sensation. The most appropriate next step is:
a Arrange a CT to define the fracture more clearly.
b Put the ankle in a cast and arrange a next-day fracture-clinic appointment.
c Reduce the fracture-dislocation under sedation in the emergency department.
d Arrange for her to have an open reduction and internal fixation on the trauma list the following day.
e Arrange for her to have a closed reduction and external fixation on the trauma list the following day.

5.5 A 43-year-old woman was brought into the emergency department by ambulance after being in a car accident. She is alert and talking to you, complaining of being short of breath. She has some bruising to the left side of her chest but no apparent limb injury, and she is not complaining of any abdominal pain. Her pulse is 120 bpm, blood pressure is 90/55 mmHg, respiratory rate is 25, and saturations are 100% on 15 L/min of oxygen. On examination, she has absent breath sounds on the left side of her chest and it is dull to percussion, with a mild tracheal shift to the right. You cannot see her JVP or any distended neck veins. Her abdomen is not distended, and it is soft and non-tender. The next course of action is:

a Place a large-bore cannula in a large vein and commence fluid resuscitation.

b Insert a chest drain into the left side of the chest.

c Arrange a chest X-ray.

d Arrange a CT of the chest and abdomen.

e Insert a large-bore cannula into the left side of the chest.

5.6 A 70-year-old man presents to you in clinic with a history of slowly progressive pain in his left knee. On examination, you notice he has a varus deformity on standing, with associated swelling of his knee and a mild effusion. He has a fixed flexion deformity and a reduced range of movement. You perform an X-ray of the left knee. You would expect to see:

a An increased joint space, subchondral sclerosis and osteophytes

b A decreased joint space with osteophytes and subchondral sclerosis

c A decreased joint space with chondrocytes and subchondral sclerosis

d An increase in joint space, osteophytes and chondrocalcinosis

e A decrease in joint space, chondrocalcinosis and chondrocytes

5.7 A 40-year-old man is brought to the emergency department by ambulance following a fall when rock climbing. He is on a spinal board, with his neck immobilised. He is complaining of some neck pain. All his observations are normal, and he has no chest, abdominal or limb injuries. With his neck immobilised, you palpate his neck and find some midline tenderness at C5. C-spine X-rays are performed with no abnormalities seen, but the body of C7 cannot be seen. The most appropriate next step is:
a Arrange a CT of the neck.
b Arrange a MRI of the neck.
c Repeat the lateral C-spine film with the arms pulled down or a swimmers view.
d Discharge the patient, as he has no C7 tenderness.
e Remove the spinal immobilisation and test the range of movement of the neck.

5.8 A 20-year-old man is admitted to the emergency department by ambulance unable to walk, smelling of alcohol and complaining of severe pain in his feet after jumping from a high wall for a dare. On examination, he has bilateral swelling and bruising of his ankles and feet, but there is no neurovascular deficit. He is maximally tender over his heels bilaterally. The rest of the exam of his lower limbs is unremarkable. The most appropriate next step is:
a Bilateral hip X-rays
b Examination of the spine
c CT scan of the feet
d Bilateral knee X-rays
e Blood alcohol level test

5.9 A 25-year-old man presents with a painful swollen knee following a bad tackle during a game of football. He says that his knee became swollen almost immediately. He also describes a feeling of instability in his knee when walking. On examination, you notice a grossly swollen knee with a large effusion. Flexion and extension are painful and are limited by the swelling in his knee. There doesn't appear to be any instability on varus or valgus stressing. The posterior drawer test is negative, but there is instability with the anterior drawer test. The knee X-ray shows a haemarthrosis. The most likely diagnosis is:
 a Lateral collateral ligament tear
 b Anterior cruciate ligament tear
 c Medial meniscal tear
 d Posterior cruciate ligament tear
 e Tibial plateau fracture

5.10 A 43-year-old man is involved in a high-speed head-on collision. He is brought into the emergency department by ambulance. He is complaining of chest discomfort and has some bruising to his chest. He appears very distressed. His heart rate is 135 bpm, blood pressure is 70/50 mmHg, respiratory rate is 25 and saturations are 100% on 15 L/min of oxygen. Examination reveals dilated neck veins, a central trachea, equal expansion of the chest, normal resonant percussion on the chest bilaterally with normal breath sounds but muffled heart sounds. You should:
 a Insert a large-bore cannula to the second intercostal space, mid-clavicular line bilaterally.
 b Arrange a chest X-ray.
 c Arrange a cardiac echo.
 d Do an ECG.
 e Perform immediate needle pericardiocentesis.

5.11 An 82-year-old woman falls while out shopping. She is brought into A&E complaining of left groin pain. She is noted to have a shortened externally rotated leg. X-ray shows a displaced intracapsular neck-of-femur fracture. The most appropriate management is:
 a Bed rest
 b Hemiarthroplasty
 c Total hip replacement
 d Traction
 e Dynamic hip screw (DHS)

5.12 An elderly man slips on ice while walking his dog and falls onto an outstretched wrist. He attends the emergency department complaining of pain in his wrist. On examination, he has a dinner-fork deformity of his wrist. The most likely diagnosis is:
  a Scaphoid fracture
  b Radial head fracture
  c Colles' fracture
  d Smith's fracture
  e Barton's fracture

5.13 A 45-year-old man attends the emergency department complaining of severe pain behind his right ankle and being unable to walk. He has just been playing squash, and he felt a snap when accelerating to get to the ball. On examination, he has swelling and bruising behind his ankle. You perform a Simmonds' test and find it to be positive. The most likely diagnosis is:
  a Ruptured Achilles' tendon
  b Ruptured deltoid ligament
  c Rupture of the posterior tibialis tendon
  d Rupture of the medial belly of gastrocnemius muscle
  e Medial malleolus fracture

5.14 A 34-year-old man has a high-speed motorbike accident in which he suffers a mid-shaft fracture of his right tibia. As the fracture is non-displaced, he is treated with immobilisation in a plaster back slab. Twelve hours following his injury, he begins to complain of excruciating pain in his leg. You cut the bandages of the back slab, but this does not improve the pain. On examination, you note that he has altered sensation in his foot and that passive movement of his ankle causes extreme pain. You diagnose compartment syndrome. The appropriate course of action is:
  a Increase his analgesia and review him in an hour.
  b Arrange a CT of his leg to assess the fracture.
  c Arrange an MRI to assess the muscles.
  d Take him to theatre and perform a fasciotomy.
  e Suggest bed rest and leg elevation.

5.15 A 65-year-old gardener with a history of gout presents to the emergency department with a painful left knee. He is complaining of being unable to flex his knee without severe pain. On examination, he has a very red and swollen knee. It has a tense effusion, and any passive movement causes extreme pain. You note that he has a temperature and on further questioning find out that he pricked his knee on a rose thorn a few days ago. You suspect a septic arthritis. The most appropriate next step is:

a Take him to theatre immediately to wash out the knee.

b Aspirate the effusion and send it for urgent Gram stain and microscopy.

c Admit him to the ward and arrange for analgesia and antibiotics.

d Send him home with a course of antibiotics.

e Organise an ultrasound scan to confirm the effusion.

5.16 A 50-year-old woman presents with pain and numbness in her right hand, and she says that it is worse at night. She describes the pain as extending up the forearm, but the numbness is only present in the hand. On examination, you notice some wasting of the thenar muscles, sensory loss over the palmer aspect of the first three-and-a-half fingers and weakness of abduction, flexion and opposition of the thumb. There is no weakness of the flexor muscles in the forearm. The most likely diagnosis is:

a Rheumatoid arthritis of the thumb

b Ulnar nerve compression at the elbow

c Median nerve compression at the wrist

d Osteoarthritis of the thumb

e Median nerve compression at the elbow

5.17 A 32-year-old man attends the orthopaedic clinic following an injury sustained while paying football. He is complaining of pain and swelling of his left knee and of not being able to straighten it. He sustained the injury when changing direction. The pain was instantaneous but the swelling did not develop immediately. Since the injury, he has been unable to straighten his knee, as he feels it is locking. You examine his knee and find a moderate-sized effusion. He has full flexion but is unable to extend his knee actively or passively. All the ligaments are intact. What is the definitive treatment for this injury?

  a MRI of the knee
  b CT of the knee
  c X-ray of the knee
  d Arthroscopy
  e Aspiration of the effusion

5.18 A 50-year-old man is brought into the emergency department by ambulance after coming off his motorbike in wet conditions. He is alert and orientated and is complaining of pain in his hips. His pulse is 120 bpm, blood pressure is 80/60 mmHg and saturations are 100% on 15 L/min of oxygen. He has good and equal air entry bilaterally. On examining his abdomen, you do not notice any distension; however, you do notice bruising to his lower abdomen and pelvis. His abdomen is soft, and the only tenderness is over the lower abdomen. You examine his pelvis and notice that his pelvic bones are mobile. You suspect an open-book pelvic fracture. The most appropriate next step is:

  a Attempt to close the pelvis with external fixator.
  b Arrange C-spine, chest and pelvis X-rays.
  c Examine the head and extremities for other injuries.
  d Gain IV access and initiate fluid resuscitation.
  e FAST (focused assessment with sonography for trauma) scan the abdomen.

5.19 A 67-year-old woman attends the orthopaedic outpatient clinic complaining of a painful shoulder. On examination, she has a painful arc of movement (70–100°). You suspect a rotator cuff tear. Which is the most common rotator cuff muscle to be torn?

  a Infraspinatus
  b Supraspinatus
  c Subscapularis
  d Teres minor
  e Teres major

5.20 A 73-year-old man presents with a very painful, acutely swollen, erythematous right knee. He has a history of gout. You want to confirm the diagnosis. The appropriate course of action is:
  a Aspirate the knee to confirm the presence of calcium pyrophosphate crystal.
  b Check serum uric acid levels.
  c Aspirate the knee, and under microscopy confirm the presence of positively birefringent crystals.
  d Begin a course of non-steroidal anti-inflammatory drugs (NSAIDs) and monitor response.
  e Perform an MRI of the knee.

5.21 Following a wrist injury, a patient presents with features of a claw hand. He has generalised wasting of the hand, with sparing of the thenar eminence. In particular, he has wasting of the first web space. On examination, he has loss of sensation over the little finger and the medial half of the fourth finger, along with the medial half of the palmer and dorsal surfaces of the hand. The findings are in keeping with:
  a Carpel tunnel syndrome
  b Radial nerve palsy
  c Diabetic neuropathy
  d Ulnar nerve palsy
  e Median nerve palsy

5.22 An overweight 14-year-old prepubescent boy complains of hip pain following playing rugby at school. He attends clinic, and you notice as he walks through the door that he has a waddling gait. On examination, the leg is externally rotated and slightly shortened. The likely diagnosis is:
  a Perthes' disease
  b Fractured neck of femur
  c Osgood-Schlatter disease
  d Slipped upper femoral epiphysis (SUFE)
  e Congenital hip dysplasia

5.23 A 48-year-old carpet layer attends clinic complaining of a painful, swollen knee. On examination, he has a swelling over his patella but no joint effusion. It is tender and hot. He has slight reduction in flexion of his knee due to pain. He has no instability of his knee on examination. He feels generally well. The likely diagnosis is:

a Prepatellar bursitis

b Septic arthritis

c Osteoarthritis

d Rheumatoid arthritis

e Baker's cyst

5.24 A 19-year-old man attends the emergency department with a painful right shoulder following an injury playing rugby. He complains of pain over his shoulder and a limited range of movement. You notice that he has a visible deformity in the line of his collarbone to his shoulder. The most likely diagnosis is:

a Rotator cuff tear

b Acromioclavicular joint disruption/dislocation

c Fracture of the humeral head

d Sternoclavicular joint disruption/dislocation

e Biceps muscle tear

5.25 A 44-year-old woman is involved in a road traffic accident and is brought to the emergency department by ambulance. She is distressed and complaining that she cannot breathe. She has visible bruising to her chest. Pulse is 110 bpm, blood pressure is 100/60 mmHg, saturations are 80% on 15 L/min of oxygen and respiratory rate is 30. She is not expanding the right side of her chest, and her trachea is deviated to the left. She is dull to percussion on the right side of her chest, with absent breath sounds on the right. The most appropriate next step is:

a Call the cardiothoracic registrar.

b Insert a large cannula to the left antecubital fossa and begin fluid resuscitation.

c X-ray the chest.

d Insert a large chest drain into the right side of the chest.

e Examine the abdomen for injuries.

5.26 A 35-year-old man sustains a blow to the head following a pub brawl. On admission, he is confused, opens his eyes to speech and withdraws in response to pain. His Glasgow Coma Score is:

a 7
b 13
c 12
d 11
e 9

5.27 A 25-year-old man is playing cricket and is struck on the side of his head by a cricket ball. Immediately following the incident, he feels well. It is unclear whether he lost consciousness for a few seconds at the time of injury. He is brought to A&E later in the day, confused, vomiting and complaining of a headache. The most likely diagnosis is:

a Concussion
b Extradural haematoma
c Meningitis
d Subdural haematoma
e Ruptured berry aneurysm

5.28 A 70-year-old man is brought to A&E by a neighbour. He has a three-week history of worsening headache, increasing confusion and unsteadiness on his feet. No clear history of trauma can be elicited; however, the patient lives on his own. He has a prosthetic heart valve and is on warfarin. The most appropriate investigation is:

a Lumbar puncture
b EEG
c CT scan brain
d Carotid duplex
e Observation

5.29 Indications for CT scanning following traumatic head injury include all of the following, EXCEPT:

a Glasgow Coma Score (GCS) <15 two hours post-injury
b Headache
c Seizure
d >1 episode of vomiting
e Focal neurology

5.30 The most common intracranial tumour in adults is:
a Medulloblastoma
b Meningioma
c Acoustic neuroma
d Metastases
e Glioma

5.31 A 22-year-old woman is seen in A&E complaining of sudden onset of a severe occipital headache. This is associated with nausea, vomiting and photophobia. She is otherwise fit and well. On examination, she is febrile, her blood pressure is 170/110 mmHg and her heart rate is 50 bpm. She has a positive Kernig's sign and third nerve palsy, and fundoscopy reveals globular subhyaloid and vitreous haemorrhages. The most likely diagnosis is:
a Subdural haematoma
b Subarachnoid haemorrhage
c Meningitis
d Encephalitis
e Meningioma

5.32 Berry aneurysms may be associated with the following conditions, EXCEPT:
a Tuberous sclerosis
b α-1 antitrypsin deficiency
c Marfan's disease
d Neurofibromatosis type 2
e Pseudoxanthoma elasticum

5.33 A 25-year-old male motorcyclist skids on ice and comes off his bike at a speed of 20 mph (32 km/h). His GCS at the scene and on admission is 15. On arrival, his blood pressure is 115/80 mmHg, heart rate is 90 bpm and saturations are 99% on room air. Examination reveals marked tenderness within the left upper quadrant and over the lower-left ribs. Blood tests demonstrate an Hb of 13.0 g/dL. Chest X-ray demonstrates a raised left hemidiaphragm only. The most appropriate next step is:
a Observation
b Chest drain insertion
c Repeat haemoglobin in four hours
d Laparotomy
e CT scan of the abdomen

5.34 A 35-year-old man is involved in a head on collision at a speed of 50 mph (80 km/h). On admission, he is intubated. His blood pressure is 80/35 mmHg and heart rate is 120 bpm. Abdominal examination is unequivocal. A diagnostic peritoneal lavage (DPL) is performed. Indications for laparotomy based on DPL findings include all of the following, EXCEPT:

a >500 000 white blood cells/mL

b Presence of stool

c Amylase >175 IU

d Frank blood on initial aspiration

e >100 000 red blood cells/mL

5.35 A 24-year-old man is involved in an altercation in a nightclub and is stabbed in the abdomen. On admission, his GCS is 14/15, blood pressure is 100/50 mmHg and heart rate is 110 bpm. Abdominal examination reveals a 2-inch (5-cm) stab wound in the iliac fossa and generalised guarding and pain. No other injuries are noted. The most appropriate next step is:

a Diagnostic peritoneal lavage

b Laparotomy

c FAST scan

d Observation

e CT scan of the abdomen

5.36 Which of the following statements is true regarding imaging in trauma?

a A trauma series consists of X-ray of the chest and AP and lateral X-rays of the cervical spine only.

b A FAST scan is useful for excluding bowel injury.

c Diagnostic peritoneal lavage is more sensitive than CT scanning for evaluating retroperitoneal injury.

d A FAST scan is superior to chest X-ray for detecting haemothorax.

e All of the above.

5.37 A 36-year-old man is stabbed multiple times in the right side of his chest. On arrival in A&E, his blood pressure is 60/15 mmHg, his heart rate is 120 bpm and he is tachypnoeic. Examination of the chest reveals decreased chest expansion, reduced breath sounds and dullness to percussion in the mid-lower zones on the right side. Chest X-ray demonstrates a large right haemothorax. A chest drain is inserted at the right fifth intercostal space in the anterior mid-axillary line, and 1600 mL of frank blood is drained. The most appropriate next step, in addition to aggressive fluid resuscitation, is:

a Thoracotomy
b Repeat chest X-ray
c CT scan of the chest
d Clamp the chest drain
e Pericardiocentesis

5.38 A seven-year-old boy is seen in clinic with a history over a few weeks of a limp and knee pain. On examination, he has a Trendelenburg gait and there is a restricted range of movement at the right hip and shortening of the right leg. The most appropriate next test is:

a X-ray of the hip and pelvis
b Arthroscopy of the hip
c MRI of the hip
d Ultrasound scan of the hip
e X-ray of the knee

5.39 Which of the following statements is true regarding congenital developmental dysplasia of the hip (DDH)?

a Boys are more commonly affected.
b It is associated with breech presentation.
c The right hip is preferentially affected.
d Family history is not important.
e Polyhydramnios is a risk factor.

5.40 The organism most commonly implicated in septic arthritis in children is:

a *Pseudomonas aeruginosa*
b *Escherichia coli*
c *Neisseria meningitidis*
d *Staphylococcus aureus*
e *Neisseria gonorrhoea*

5.41 A 35-year-old man falls onto an outstretched hand and complains of discomfort in his wrist. Examination reveals exquisite tenderness in the anatomical snuffbox; there is no deformity or limitation in range of wrist movement. X-ray of the wrist does not demonstrate any abnormality. The most appropriate next step is:
a Reassure and discharge
b Physiotherapy
c MRI of the wrist
d Repeat X-ray of the wrist at two weeks
e Surgical exploration of the wrist joint

5.42 Which of the following statements is true regarding shoulder dislocations?
a Inferior dislocations of the shoulder are more common.
b In anterior dislocation, the arm is held abducted and externally rotated.
c There is a higher risk of damage to the axillary nerve with posterior dislocations.
d Associated rotator cuff injury is seen to be greater in younger patients.
e X-ray of the shoulder joint is not required following reduction of the dislocation.

5.43 A 37-year-old man has been in a below-knee plaster cast for management of an ankle fracture for six weeks. On removal of the cast, he complains of numbness in the leg and cannot hold his foot horizontal. On examination, he has foot drop and altered sensation over the lateral aspect of the calf and dorsum of the foot. His symptoms are most likely to be due to:
a Cauda equina syndrome
b Sciatic nerve injury
c Tibial nerve injury
d Common peroneal nerve injury
e Popliteal nerve injury

5.44 In the case of blunt chest trauma in a haemodynamically stable patient, if the chest X-ray demonstrates a widened mediastinum, the most appropriate next diagnostic investigation would be:
a FAST ultrasound scan
b ECG
c Lateral chest X-ray
d CT angiogram of the chest
e Nothing, but observe

5.45 The following are causes of a widened mediastinum on chest radiograph, EXCEPT:
a Sarcoidosis
b Thymoma
c Hodgkin's lymphoma
d Non-Hodgkin's lymphoma
e Amyloidosis

ANSWERS

5.1   The correct answer is C.

The clinical signs of tachycardia, hypotension, raised JVP/prominent neck veins, hypoxia, tracheal deviation away from the side of injury, hyper-resonance and lack of breath sounds are classical for a tension pneumothorax. The most appropriate course of action, therefore, is insertion of a large-bore cannula into the right side of the chest (second intercostal space, midclavicular line) to decompress the tension pneumothorax, following which a chest drain will need to be inserted.

5.2   The correct answer is B.

The radial nerve lies against the mid-shaft of the humerus in the radial/spiral groove and is susceptible to damage in fractures of the mid-shaft of the humerus. To test for damage to the radial nerve, you can test sensation over the anatomical snuffbox and extensor surface of the forearm, and you can test motor function by examining the wrist/finger extensors.

5.3   The correct answer is D.

The clinical presentation of back pain with reduced power in the lower legs and absent ankle reflexes, altered perianal/perineal sensation and urinary retention is indicative of a cauda equina compression. In this case, it may be secondary to metastatic breast cancer. MRI is the investigation of choice to assess for compression of the spinal cord. This needs to be done urgently, as, if not treated, irreversible damage can be done.

5.4   The correct answer is C.

If there is evidence of vascular compromise following an ankle fracture-dislocation, it is important to reduce the fracture-dislocation immediately.

5.5   The correct answer is A.

The clinical picture suggests that the patient has a left-sided haemothorax. As she is maintaining her saturations and she is in hypovolaemic shock, she needs IV access and the commencement of fluids prior to the insertion of a chest drain.

5.6   The correct answer is B.

The history suggests osteoarthritis of the knee joint. The classical X-ray signs of osteoarthritis are a reduced joint space, osteophytes, subchondral sclerosis, bone cysts and chondrocalcinosis.

5.7   The correct answer is C.

You cannot clear a C-spine if there is any spinal tenderness without having radiological imaging of the whole C-spine. If the body of C7 cannot be seen on a normal lateral, simply pulling the arms towards the feet may be enough to visualise it. If not, a 'swimmers view' can be performed to visualise the lower C-spine. These simple manoeuvres can prevent unnecessary CT scanning. However, if there is any doubt, a CT scan should be performed.

5.8   The correct answer is B.

The history and examination is highly suggestive of bilateral calcaneal fractures. The mechanism of injury and the force required to cause bilateral calcaneal fractures can result in compression fracture of the spine. Up to 10–15% of people suffering calcaneal fracture will have associated spinal compression fractures.

5.9   The correct answer is B.

The anterior drawer test tests the anterior cruciate ligament. The valgus stress test tests the medial collateral and the varus stress test tests the lateral collateral. The posterior drawer test tests the posterior cruciate. A meniscal tear is unlikely to cause a haemarthrosis, and you would not bear weight with a tibial plateau fracture.

5.10   The correct answer is E.

The history suggests severe blunt chest trauma. The clinical signs are in keeping with cardiac tamponade, and therefore decompression of the pericardium is essential. Cardiac tamponade presents similarly to a tension pneumothorax. However, with the tension pneumothorax you do not get muffled heart sounds; you do get absent breath sounds and hyper-resonance on the affected side with tracheal deviation.

5.11   The correct answer is B.

Intracapsular fractures have a high risk of avascular necrosis of the head of the femur if they are displaced; therefore a hemiarthroplasty should be performed. Non-displaced intracapsular fractures can be fixed with internal fixation screws. Extracapsular fractures can be fixed with a DHS.

5.12 The correct answer is C.

A Colles' fracture is a fracture of the distal radius, with dorsal angulation of the distal fragment causing the classic dinner-fork deformity. It is commonly caused by falling onto an outstretched hand. Smith's and Barton's fractures are also fractures of the wrist, but they do not cause the dinner-fork deformity. An isolated scaphoid fracture doesn't cause deformity. The radial head fracture is an elbow fracture.

5.13 The correct answer is A.

The history is classical of an Achilles' tendon rupture. Simmonds' test is done by getting the patient to kneel on a chair and then squeezing the calf, which would normally cause planter flexion of the foot. However, when the Achilles' tendon is ruptured, you do not see any movement. This is a positive Simmonds' test.

5.14 The correct answer is D.

Once compartment syndrome has been diagnosed, the only course of treatment is to relieve pressure within the compartment; this means a fasciotomy. As the severe pain is being caused by muscle ischaemia, any unnecessary delay can result in muscle loss.

5.15 The correct answer is B.

You should confirm the diagnosis of septic arthritis by aspirating the effusion and sending it for urgent microscopy. It could be that this is an episode of gout and therefore it would not be appropriate to take him straight to theatre. If it is a septic arthritis, antibiotics alone will not be enough; he will need the joint washed out.

5.16 The correct answer is C.

The symptoms are consistent with carpel tunnel syndrome. This is caused by compression of the median nerve as it passes through the carpel tunnel at the level of the wrist. Although pain can be referred up the forearm, there is no sensory or motor dysfunction proximal to the carpel tunnel. This is what differentiates it from compression of the median nerve more proximally.

5.17 The correct answer is D.

The assessment of the patient strongly suggests a meniscal tear. Although an MRI would help in the diagnosis, it is not a definitive treatment. An arthroscopy, however, will confirm the diagnosis, and you will be able to treat/repair the injury at that time.

5.18 The correct answer is D.

The priority is to gain IV access before undertaking any further tasks, as the patient is in hypovolaemic shock due to blood loss from his pelvic fracture. Once IV access is gained and fluid resuscitation is commenced, the pelvis should be closed to reduce potential space for blood loss and to tamponade the bleeding.

5.19 The correct answer is C.

The subscapularis is the most common muscle to be torn in rotator cuff injuries, resulting in difficulties in initiating abduction. All the muscles named above, except teres major, are rotator cuff muscles.

5.20 The correct answer is C.

Calcium pyrophosphate crystals are found in pseudogout; it is uric acid (urate) crystals that cause gout, and these are positively birefringent on microscopy. Although plasma uric acid may be high during attacks of gout, it doesn't exclude septic arthritis as the cause of the painful knee.

5.21 The correct answer is D.

The features are classical of ulnar nerve palsy. The patient will also exhibit weakness of the interossei and abductor digiti minimi.

5.22 The correct answer is D.

SUFE commonly occurs in overweight prepubescent boys. It doesn't always occur following injury, but acute slips often do. It can also present with knee pain due to the hip pain being referred. Diagnosis is made by X-ray showing slippage of the epiphysis.

5.23 The correct answer is A.

Prepatellar bursitis is an occupational hazard of carpet fitting and other professions that involve kneeling a lot. The treatment is to avoid exacerbating activity, firm bandaging, NSAIDs and aspiration if indicated.

5.24 The correct answer is B.

Acromioclavicular disruption/dislocation is most common in males in their second decade, and it is a common injury in rugby due to going into tackle with the shoulder first. It causes a step between the acromion and clavicle, resulting in deformity.

5.25 The correct answer is D.

The clinical signs are consistent with a right haemothorax. The patient has respiratory compromise and according to Advance Trauma Life Support (ATLS©) guidelines, B (breathing) should be dealt with immediately before progressing to C (circulation).

5.26 The correct answer is D.

The Glasgow Coma Score (GCS) is an objective method of assessing a patient neurologically, and it assesses best eye, verbal and motor responses:

- Eyes opening: 4 = spontaneous, 3 = to command, 2 = to pain, 1 = none
- Verbal response: 5 = orientated, 4 = confused, 3 = inappropriate words, 2 = incomprehensible sounds, 1 = none
- Motor response: 6 = obeys commands, 5 = localises to pain, 4 = withdraws from pain, 3 = abnormal flexion to pain, 2 = extension to pain, 1 = none.

5.27 The correct answer is B.

An extradural haematoma is a neurosurgical emergency. It typically occurs as a result of a bleed from the middle meningeal artery, commonly associated with a linear fracture of the squamous temporal bone. Classically, there is an initial loss of consciousness followed by a lucid interval then a decline in consciousness.

5.28 The correct answer is C.

The patient has a history suggestive of a chronic subdural haematoma. This commonly occurs due to tearing and bleeding from the bridging veins, which are more fragile in the elderly. Often a history of trauma is forgotten, as it may be trivial; however, subdural haematomas can occur spontaneously in patients on anticoagulants/antiplatelets. Other risk factors include age (they usually occur in people in their 60s and 70s), alcoholism and coagulopathy.

5.29 The correct answer is B.

Indications for immediate CT scanning of the brain following traumatic head injury are outlined in the guidelines *Head Injury – Triage, assessment, investigation and early management of head injury in infants, children and adults: NICE Clinical Guideline 56* (2007). These include GCS <13 on presentation, GCS <15 two hours post-injury, suspected skull fracture, signs of basal skull fracture, seizure, focal neurology, >1 episode of vomiting, and amnesia for events >30 minutes prior to event.

5.30 The correct answer is E.

Gliomas account for approximately 50% of all brain tumours in adults; metastases and meningiomas account for approximately 15% each. Symptoms are due to a combination of increased intracranial pressure and compression/mass effects.

5.31 The correct answer is B.

Headache, nausea and vomiting, and hypertension with bradycardia (Cushing's response) are due to increased intracranial pressure. Signs of meningism are due to irritation of the meninges by blood. Third nerve palsy occurs because of compression.

5.32 The correct answer is D.

Berry aneurysms are associated with neurofibromatosis type 1. Notably, rupture of a berry aneurysm accounts for the majority of subarachnoid haemorrhages.

5.33 The correct answer is E.

The spleen is injured in approximately 25–30% of all blunt abdominal trauma. Clinical features are often subtle and include abdominal pain, referred shoulder-tip pain, abdominal distension, peritonitis and shock – the latter makes the diagnosis more obvious. Importantly, young patients may not decompensate until later. In the unstable patient, laparotomy is the management of choice, and DPL or bedside FAST ultrasound scanning of the abdomen for free intraperitoneal blood may be performed as an adjunct if abdominal signs are unequivocal and multiple other injuries are present. In the stable patient, as in this case, CT scanning is the imaging modality of choice, although chest and abdominal radiographs may give some clues, e.g. associated lower-rib fractures, medial displacement of the gastric bubble, raised left hemidiaphragm, pleural effusion.

5.34 The correct answer is A.

DPL is a sensitive and specific test for evaluating intra-abdominal injury in the unstable trauma patient, where CT scanning is contraindicated.

A positive DPL result includes: 10 mL of blood or enteric contents on initial aspiration, >100 000 red blood cells/mL (>10 000 red blood cells/mL in penetrating trauma), >500 white blood cells/mL and amylase >175 IU.

5.35 The correct answer is B.

Shock, peritonitis and evisceration are all indications for urgent laparotomy in penetrating trauma. If these are absent, FAST scanning or DPL is advised; if these are negative, the patient should be admitted and observed, and laparoscopy or CT scanning may be performed the following day.

5.36 The correct answer is D.

A trauma series consists of a lateral X-ray of the C-spine and AP X-rays of the chest and pelvis. FAST exam is useful and highly sensitive for evaluating free fluid within the peritoneal, pericardial and pleural cavities. It is also thought to be equally or more sensitive than chest X-ray for evaluating haemo- and pneumothorax; approximately 200 mL of fluid needs to be present in the pleural cavity to be detected on chest X-ray, and approximately 50 mL needs to be present with FAST scan. CT scanning of the abdomen is superior to ultrasound for demonstrating soft-tissue injury, bowel injury and retroperitoneal injury. DPL, although sensitive and specific for intra-abdominal injury in blunt trauma, is not useful for retroperitoneal bleeding.

5.37 The correct answer is A.

The patient has a massive haemothorax. Penetrating trauma has an increased likelihood of being associated with arterial bleeding that is less likely to settle compared to venous bleeding. Thoracomy is indicated if, as in this case, the immediate drain output is >1000–1500 mL or there is >200–250 mL drained in three consecutive hours.

5.38 The correct answer is A.

The patient has Perthes' disease, which is avascular necrosis of the proximal femoral head. It is more common in boys between the ages of 4 and 10 years. Presentation may be with a limp; limited range of movements of the hip; pain within the hip (often referred to the thigh or knee), which may be worse with passive movement and fixed flexion; external rotation and adduction deformities of the leg; and leg shortening. The aetiology is unknown. X-ray of the hip and pelvis (AP and frog lateral views) will aid diagnosis, and in advanced stages there is collapse of the femoral head, causing it to appear widened and flattened. Full blood count and ESR should also be performed to exclude septic causes.

5.39 The correct answer is B.

DDH is instability or dysplasia of the hip joint. It is more common in girls and firstborns. The left hip is affected three times more often that the right hip. DDH is associated with breech presentation, oligohydramnios, multiple gestations, and other congenital abnormalities (e.g. club foot and torticollis). Children of parents with DDH and subsequent siblings are at increased risk of developing DDH. Presentation is usually in neonatal life. Ortolani's manoeuvre and Barlow's test demonstrate reducible or irreducible dislocation and subluxation, respectively, and form part of neonatal screening.

5.40 The correct answer is D.

Septic arthritis is a medical emergency. The most common organism implicated is *Staphylococcus aureus* in all age groups; group B *Streptococcus* is the next most common pathogen. Of note, *Haemophilus influenzae*, prior to the introduction of the Hib vaccination, used to be implicated in the majority of cases of septic arthritis in those under three years old. *Neisseria gonorrhoea* may be acquired from an infected birth canal in neonates and is a common cause in young adults. The other organisms listed in the question may also cause septic arthritis.

5.41 The correct answer is D.

Diagnosis of scaphoid fractures is usually by X-ray of the wrist. However, if the fracture is not displaced, X-rays performed immediately may not demonstrate the fracture. Patients with significant pain over the anatomical snuffbox should be treated as having a scaphoid fracture and splinted, with repeat X-ray performed at two weeks. CT and MRI of the wrist may be useful for assessing for a fracture in selected cases. Non-displaced scaphoid fractures are treated by immobilisation in a cast for six weeks. Displaced fractures require surgical fixation with screws or pins. Complications of scaphoid fractures include non-union, avascular necrosis (typically of the proximal third) and early arthritis.

5.42 The correct answer is B.

Anterior dislocations account for the majority of shoulder dislocations. It has a bimodal distribution and occurs in young adults typically due to sporting injuries and in the elderly due to falls. Risk of damage to the axillary nerve is greatest with anterior dislocations; therefore you should assess sensation over the 'regimental patch' distribution of the arm and deltoid function. In posterior dislocations the arm is held adducted and internally rotated; and neurovascular compromise is not often seen. Associated rotator cuff injury is seen typically in older patients. Pre- and post-reduction X-ray of the shoulder should be performed (to assess for associated fractures/pathology). In addition, assessment should be made for neurovascular compromise.

5.43 The correct answer is D.

The common peroneal nerve is a terminal branch of the sciatic nerve (which divides in the popliteal fossa to form the tibial and common peroneal nerves) and is derived from L4, L5, S1 and S2 nerve roots. The common peroneal nerve itself divides to form the superficial and deep peroneal nerves. The superficial peroneal nerve innervates muscles of the lateral compartment of the leg (the foot evertors) and skin overlying the lateral aspect of the calf and dorsum of the foot. The deep peroneal nerve innervates muscles in the anterior compartment of the leg (the foot/toe flexors) and skin in the first and second web space. Damage to the common peroneal nerve typically occurs at the level of the head of the fibula, where it is the most superficial. Symptoms include foot drop and numbness/tingling in the aforementioned distribution.

5.44 The correct answer is D.

In blunt chest trauma, the possibility of aortic injury should always be borne in mind. Although patients with complete thoracic aorta transaction will die at the scene, those with partial tears may survive and remain relatively haemodynamically stable, at least initially. A widened mediastinum on chest X-ray has a sensitivity of approximately 50–60% for aortic injury, and a CT scan with contrast should be performed if mediastinal widening is seen in this context. Note that angiography was previously the gold-standard investigation.

5.45 The correct answer is E.

It should be noted that both Hodgkin's and non-Hodgkin's lymphoma can give rise to a widened mediastinum.

6

Perioperative and Critical Care

QUESTIONS

6.1 Two days after a sigmoid colectomy, a 65-year-old woman develops fever, rigors and oliguria as she is having a blood transfusion to correct her post-operative anaemia. What is the most appropriate course of action?

a Continue the blood transfusion, while administering paracetamol.

b Continue the blood transfusion but also prescribe regular chlorpheniramine.

c Stop the transfusion immediately and give a stat dose of intravenous hydrocortisone.

d Stop the transfusion immediately; maintain blood pressure and renal function with aggressive fluid resuscitation. Send off blood samples from both the donor unit and the recipient.

e Perform a septic screen.

6.2 A 75-year-old man had a laryngectomy and is therefore nil by mouth for at least one week. Which of the following would be the most appropriate form of nutritional support?

a Nasogastric-tube feeding

b Normal saline infusion

c Total parenteral nutrition

d Peripheral parenteral nutrition

e Hartmann's infusion

6.3 A 68-year-old woman is to be admitted in two weeks for removal of a rectal polyp as a day case. Which of her regular medications should she not take before coming to hospital?
a Atenolol
b Salbutamol inhaler
c Bendroflumethiazide
d Co-dydramol
e Glibenclamide

6.4 Vitamin K is required for the hepatic synthesis of:
a Coagulation factors III, VII, IX and X
b Coagulation factors II, VII, IX and X
c Coagulation factors II, VI, X and XI
d Coagulation factors I, VIII, X and XI
e Coagulation factors I, VII, IX and X

6.5 A 30-year-old man is diagnosed in A&E with a supraventricular tachycardia. He is otherwise well and not on any other medications. What is the treatment of choice, failing carotid massage?
a Intravenous lidocaine
b Intravenous hydrocortisone
c Intravenous digoxin
d Intravenous amiodarone
e Intravenous adenosine

6.6 Which of the following does NOT predispose to deep venous thrombosis (DVT)?
a Recent surgery
b Obesity
c Age <60 years
d Immobility
e Malignancy

6.7 A 50-year-old man is found to have persistently high blood pressure, measuring 190/110 mmHg. He also complains of periodic headaches but denies any chest pain or breathlessness. Clinical examination is unremarkable; however, his ECG demonstrates ST segment depression in the left ventricular leads. What is the best management plan?

a Admit him to hospital for intravenous antihypertensives.

b Suggest altering predisposing lifestyle factors and reassess in six months.

c Start him on a statin.

d Prescribe oral antihypertensives and reassess in three months.

e Prescribe oral antihypertensives and reassess in two weeks.

6.8 An alcoholic is admitted for an emergency appendicectomy. The day after surgery, he becomes confused, agitated and delusional. The likely diagnosis is:

a Alcoholic hallucinosis

b Wernicke's encephalopathy

c Korsakoff's syndrome

d Delirium tremens

e Adverse drug reaction

6.9 Which of the following statements is NOT true of abdominal laparoscopic surgery?

a There is evidence of quicker recovery periods post-operatively.

b Earlier discharge is associated with laparoscopic surgery.

c Laparoscopic operations tend to be shorter.

d Wounds are smaller in laparoscopic-assisted procedures.

e A general anaesthetic is always required.

6.10 A reduced ratio of forced expiratory volume in one second to forced vital capacity is characteristic of which condition?

a Pulmonary fibrosis

b Kyphoscoliosis

c Pleural effusion

d Chronic obstructive pulmonary disease

e Polio

6.11 The most common cause of oliguric renal failure in post-operative patients is:
a Adverse drug reaction
b Hypovolaemia
c Sepsis
d Blood transfusion
e Blocked urinary catheter

6.12 A 74-year-old male patient on the surgical ward has a central venous line placed for intravenous feeding. Immediately following the procedure, he begins to feel short of breath and his oxygen saturations fall. The most likely diagnosis is:
a Air embolism
b Expanding haematoma in the neck
c Pneumothorax
d Myocardial infarction
e Chest infection

6.13 An insulin-dependent diabetic patient on the ward becomes aggressive, and on examination, he is sweaty, incoherent and tachycardic. His BM reads 2.2 mmol/L. How would you treat this patient?
a Give him stat IV dexamethasone.
b Administer 20 mL 20% dextrose IV fast.
c Administer 50 mL 100% dextrose IV fast.
d Administer 50 mL 50% dextrose IV fast.
e Give him 2 mg IM glucagon.

6.14 A 45-year-old female patient suddenly becomes short of breath and collapses on the ward 10 days following her surgery. The likely diagnosis is a pulmonary embolism. What findings do you look for on the ECG?
a Sinus tachycardia
b Sinus bradycardia
c S-waves in II, Q-waves in I and inverted T-waves in I
d S-waves in I, Q-waves in II and inverted T-waves in III
e S-waves in I, Q-waves in III and inverted T-waves in III

6.15 A young man is admitted to hospital following a road traffic accident while riding his motorcycle. His only injury is a compound right femoral shaft fracture. What is his estimated blood loss from this fracture?
a 150 mL
b 1500 mL
c 2000 mL
d 3000 mL
e 3500 mL

6.16 A young woman presents to preassessment clinic, and on direct questioning she admits to symptoms of thirst, polyuria, weight loss and recurrent episodes of thrush. What single investigation will confirm your diagnosis?
a Full blood count
b Fasting blood glucose
c Urine dipstick
d High vaginal swab
e Serum ADH

6.17 A 65-year-old female surgical patient with a history of ischaemic heart disease suddenly collapses on the ward and becomes unresponsive. She has no carotid pulse, so basic cardiopulmonary resuscitation (CPR) is commenced. A cardiac monitor then shows ventricular fibrillation (VF). What should you do?
a Give 3 mg adrenaline IV.
b Continue with basic life support.
c Defibrillation with 500 J (monophasic).
d Defibrillation with 360 J (monophasic).
e Give 300 mg amiodarone IV.

6.18 A known epileptic is admitted to a surgical ward following minor surgery. All his observations are fine until he suddenly starts to fit uncontrollably. After securing his airway, gaining IV access and ensuring that his BM is normal, what would be the next course of action?
a Call the anaesthetist.
b Give 1 mg diazepam IV.
c Give 50 mL 50% dextrose IV.
d Give 50 mg phenytoin IV.
e Give 4 mg lorazepam IV.

6.19 A 75-year-old male surgical patient begins to complain of a painful great toe several days following his surgery. His serum urate levels are high, and an X-ray of his foot is normal. What would you give him to relieve this acute attack?
a Co-dydramol
b Naproxen
c Probenecid
d Colchicine
e Allopurinol

6.20 A 90-year-old female patient becomes acutely short of breath, coughing up frothy sputum, three days after an emergency laparotomy. Her oxygen saturations are low at 80%. She is dyspnoeic and tachycardic, and on chest examination, she has widespread wheeze. After sitting her up and giving her oxygen by face mask, what would you do?
a Give diamorphine IM.
b Organise a routine chest X-ray.
c Give her GTN spray.
d Give furosemide 40–80 mg IV.
e Give a salbutamol nebuliser.

6.21 A 45-year-old previously fit and healthy man is back on the ward following a Hartmann's procedure for a perforated sigmoid tumour. His blood pressure has been gradually falling over the last two hours, and his pulse rate is rising. His urine output over the past hour is zero, and there is minimal output from his abdominal drains. Which of the following statements regarding this patient is correct?
a Post-operative bleeding is unlikely as there is minimal abdominal-drain output.
b The patient is in hypovolaemic shock.
c The urinary catheter is probably blocked.
d CVP monitoring is unlikely to help guide fluid resuscitation.
e An urgent CT scan of the abdomen should be performed.

6.22 A 75-year-old man becomes unwell four days following a right hemicolectomy for colon cancer. He is complaining of feeling very short of breath and very hot. His observations show a heart rate of 110 bpm, blood pressure of 100/60 mmHg, respiratory rate of 30 and saturations of 91% on 15 L/min of oxygen. Bloods show a white cell count of 18 and C-reactive protein of 350. On examination, he looks very unwell and tired. On auscultation, he has bronchial breathing at the right base. Chest X-ray demonstrates shadowing of the right lower zone. You perform an arterial blood gas, which shows a pH of 7.25, PaO_2 of 7.8 kPa and pCO_2 of 6.5 kPa. You suspect a post-op chest infection. The most appropriate next step is:

a Start oral antibiotics and organise chest physiotherapy.

b Start IV antibiotics and saline nebs and chest physiotherapy.

c Give him a bolus of IV fluid and start IV antibiotics.

d Give him a bolus of IV fluid and IV antibiotics; catheterise him and call the ITU registrar with a view to CPAP/intubation.

e Start intravenous antibiotics.

6.23 A 77-year-old woman becomes more unwell on HDU 12 hours following a Hartmann's procedure for a perforated sigmoid diverticulum. You are asked to see her because her blood pressure and urine output are low. She has a heart rate of 115 bpm, a blood pressure of 80/40 mmHg, saturations of 95% on 40% inspired oxygen, a urine output of 20 mL for the last two hours and a temperature of 38.2 °C. She looks unwell and is slightly drowsy. However, she has warm peripheries. You prescribe 500 mL of Gelofusin (a synthetic colloid) stat, which has very little effect on her blood pressure, and you then give another 500 mL. She has a slight improvement in blood pressure to 90/40 mmHg but is not passing any urine. A CVP line is inserted, and CVP is 12. A further 250 mL of Gelofusin is given, and CVP rises to 13. Her blood pressure is still 90/40 mmHg, and there is no urine output. The most appropriate next step is:

a Give a further 500 mL and review in an hour.

b Do not give any more boluses, but increase fluids to 1 L over four hours.

c Continue eight-hourly fluids as CVP 13.

d Consider ionotropes.

e Start GTN infusion.

6.24 A 74-year-old woman with a history of myocardial infarction (MI) develops acute shortness of breath two days following a laparotomy for an obstruction sigmoid tumour. She denies any chest pain. Her observations show a heart rate of 95 bpm, blood pressure of 120/85 mmHg, saturations of 92% on 40% inspired oxygen and a respiratory rate of 25. On auscultation, she has bilateral crepitations to the mid-zone, and you notice she has a degree of peripheral oedema. You perform an arterial blood gas, which shows pH 7.38, pO_2 7.8 kPa and pCO_2 5 kPa. No acute changes are seen on her ECG. The most appropriate next step is:
 a Give treatment-dose Clexane for suspected pulmonary embolism.
 b Give furosemide to treat pulmonary oedema.
 c Start antibiotics for chest infection.
 d Increase the oxygen only.
 e Arrange chest physiotherapy for presumed atelectasis.

6.25 Basic life support (BLS) requires the following, EXCEPT:
 a Establishment of a definitive airway
 b 30 chest compressions to be given immediately, followed by two rescue breaths
 c Chest compressions and ventilation at a rate of 30:2
 d Leaving the casualty to summon help if necessary
 e Rescue breaths to be given over one second

6.26 A 65-year-old man who had a previous laparotomy has been admitted 24 hours ago with small-bowel obstruction (SBO) secondary to adhesion and is being treated conservatively. You are asked to see him because he has a low urine output of <30 mL/hour. His fluid balance for the last 24 hours shows him to be 1.5 L positive. His abdomen is distended but non-tender. The most appropriate next step is:
 a Give no more fluid, as he has a positive balance, and give him furosemide.
 b Increase his IV fluids and furosemide.
 c Increase his IV fluids and reassess.
 d Take him to theatre, as his SBO is not resolving.
 e Arrange a CVP line to be inserted.

6.27 During a left hemicolectomy, a 42-year-man underwent splenectomy following inadvertent damage to the spleen. In the long term, he is at greatest risk of infection from which organism?
a Mycosis fungoides
b *Streptococcus pneumoniae*
c *Clostridium difficile*
d HIV
e *Neisseria meningitidis*

6.28 Heparin exerts its anticoagulant effect through:
a Inhibition of antithrombin
b Activation of antithrombin
c Inhibition of vitamin K dependent clotting factors
d Activation of factor Xa
e Inhibition of factor VIII

6.29 The following are recognised causes of pyrexia in the post-op patient, EXCEPT:
a Atelectasis
b Blood transfusion
c Pulmonary oedema
d Pulmonary embolus
e Resolving haematoma

6.30 A 40-year-old is scheduled for elective splenectomy for hypersplenism secondary to idiopathic thrombocytopaenic purpura. Which of the following statements is correct?
a Re-vaccination for pneumococcus is recommended every five years.
b Vaccinations should ideally be administered at induction.
c Vaccinations should ideally be administered one week pre-operatively.
d Prophylactic antibiotics are recommended for five years post-operatively.
e Amoxicillin 250 mg four times daily is the recommended prophylactic dose.

6.31 A 45-year-old woman has undergone small-bowel resection for Crohn's disease. A significant amount of small bowel was diseased and resected, and a primary anastomosis between the jejunum and colon was formed. Long-term complications of surgery include the following, EXCEPT:
   a Vitamin B12 deficiency
   b Hypomagnesaemia
   c Diarrhoea
   d Jaundice
   e Renal stones

6.32 Donor blood for transfusion is routinely screened in the UK for the following, EXCEPT:
   a Chagas' disease
   b Syphilis
   c Hepatitis B
   d Hepatitis C
   e HIV

6.33 Which of the following statements is true regarding brainstem death?
   a Diagnosis should be performed by two clinicians of ≥ five years' registration, at least one of whom is a consultant.
   b Prior to diagnosis, reversible causes of coma should be excluded.
   c EEG activity may persist despite brainstem death.
   d Members of the transplant team cannot diagnose brainstem death.
   e All of the above.

6.34 A 78-year-old man is found in a house fire. On examination on arrival in hospital, he has a Glasgow Coma Score (GCS) of 14, blood pressure of 90/40 mmHg and heart rate of 100 bpm. He has singed facial hair and carbonaceous sputum. His entire right arm is painful, red and blistering. No other injuries are noted. Which of the following statements is true regarding his injuries?
   a His age will not affect his outcome.
   b He is unlikely to have sustained an inhalation injury.
   c Opiate analgesia should be avoided, as his GCS is altered.
   d He is at risk of developing hypothermia.
   e He has 18% second-degree burns.

6.35 The following factors are associated with an increased perioperative risk, EXCEPT:

a Age >60 years
b BMI <20
c Diabetes mellitus
d Previous DVT
e Renal failure

ANSWERS

6.1   The correct answer is D.

This is potentially a severe haemolytic transfusion reaction. In addition to fluid support, she may need intravenous steroids and antihistamines or even adrenaline in severe cases.

6.2   The correct answer is C.

Peripheral parenteral nutrition is more appropriate when short-term feeding (three to four days) is required.

6.3   The correct answer is E.

Oral hypoglycaemics should be omitted on the morning of minor surgery and restarted when the patient is eating normally post-operatively. Long-acting sulphonylureas need to be stopped 48 hours prior to surgery, because of the risk of hypoglycaemia perioperatively.

6.4   The correct answer is B.

6.5   The correct answer is E.

6.6   The correct answer is C.

Age >60 years is associated with a greater tendency towards DVT. A history of DVT or pulmonary embolism, pregnancy, the combined oral contraceptive pill, long-distance air travel and jaundice also predispose to DVT. The administration of subcutaneous heparin and graduated calf-compression stockings, pre- and post-operatively, has been proven to reduce the incidence of this complication.

6.7   The correct answer is E.

Two weeks is generally sufficient to see if the medication is effective or if the patient has had any side effects that could reduce compliance. If there are any issues, an alternative can be prescribed at this point rather than after waiting several months.

6.8   The correct answer is D.

This patient should have been commenced on regular chlordiazepoxide on admission in order to prevent the symptoms of alcohol withdrawal.

6.9 The correct answer is C.

Laparoscopic procedures tend to take longer, particularly at the start of the surgeon's learning curve.

6.10 The correct answer is D.

6.11 The correct answer is B.

All of the above can lead to renal failure, but it is most commonly attributed to hypovolaemia in the surgical patient, so the correct answer is B. This is particularly so post-operatively where insensible losses are not taken into account in patients who may not be able to supplement their fluid needs orally.

6.12 The correct answer is C.

The risk of air embolism is low if appropriate measures are taken prior to central-venous cannulation. Measures include having the patient head down and ensuring that the line is flushed through with saline prior to insertion. Upper-airway obstruction secondary to a haematoma within the neck is rare again but has been reported in patients with coagulopathies. Crushing central chest pain associated with shortness of breath and typical ECG changes would be suggestive of a myocardial infarction.

6.13 The correct answer is D.

The correct dose is 50–100 mL of 50% dextrose. Dexamethasone can be used in addition in cases of prolonged hypoglycaemia where there is concern about developing cerebral oedema. If you cannot gain IV access, glucagon can be given IM. Once the patient is fully conscious, he can have sugary drinks.

6.14 The correct answer is E.

However, the ECG is most commonly normal, or there is sinus tachycardia. Other features to look for include right bundle branch block and right axis deviation.

6.15 The correct answer is D.

If the fracture is closed, estimated blood losses are half of this value. Blood loss from the ribs is 150 mL, from the pelvis is 2000 mL and from tibial fractures is 650 mL, but these values are doubled if the fracture is compound.

6.16 The correct answer is B.

This patient presents with symptoms suggestive of diabetes mellitus, so the best investigation to confirm this is a fasting venous glucose, which should be greater than 7 mmol/L on two occasions. Glycosuria should prompt investigations, as above, even if the patient is symptomless.

6.17 The correct answer is D.

According to Resuscitation Council guidelines, she should be defibrillated with 360 J as soon as you have made the diagnosis of VF. CPR is immediately recommenced 30:2 for two minutes. If VF persists after two further shocks, consider giving 300 mg of amiodarone IV. One mg of adrenaline IV is given every three to five minutes throughout the resuscitation.

6.18 The correct answer is E.

Rectal diazepam can also be given if IV access is difficult. Phenytoin can be given if the seizures continue (unless the patient is already on phenytoin, when paraldehyde can be given), 50 mg/min up to a total of 1000 mg. An anaesthetist should be involved if seizures continue beyond 40 minutes, as the patient may need to be paralysed and ventilated.

6.19 The correct answer is B.

Non-steroidal anti-inflammatory drugs (NSAIDs), e.g. indomethacin, rather than opioids are indicated in the treatment of acute gout. Alternatively, colchicine can be given if there is a history of peptic ulceration. Allopurinol can be started three weeks after an acute attack to prevent future relapses.

6.20 The correct answer is D.

This is a typical presentation of acute pulmonary oedema, which is particularly common in elderly patients, who may have been fluid overloaded in the early post-operative period. An urgent chest X-ray or ECG should not precede treatment if the patient has all the clinical signs and is in extremis. Diamorphine can also be given in 1 mg intravenous boluses. Salbutamol nebulisers are helpful if the patient has cardiac wheeze.

6.21 The correct answer is B.

The patient has features of hypovolaemic shock. In the post-operative patient, a surgical bleed should be excluded. CT scanning should not be performed in a haemodynamically unstable patient.

6.22 The correct answer is D.

This patient is unwell and septic, with a high pCO_2 and high respiratory rate. These are signs that he is tiring and his ventilation and gas exchange are worsening. This patient needs urgent review by ITU, as he may very well require ventilatory support.

6.23 The correct answer is D.

This person is septic. Her blood pressure is low not because she is hypovolaemic but because she is in septic shock; this is why her peripheries are warm, not cold. More fluid may put her into pulmonary oedema, but she needs her blood pressure increased, as she is not perfusing her organs adequately (as shown by urine output). Therefore she needs inotropes, of which the first line is noradrenaline; this will bring her blood pressure up and should improve tissue perfusion.

6.24 The correct answer is B.

It is common for elderly patients to develop pulmonary oedema post-operatively. This is often due to too aggressive fluid administration and fluids should be administered more thoughtfully in the elderly patient, especially if they have a background of previous ischaemic heart disease. Treatment of pulmonary oedema should be with furosemide with or without a glycerol trinitrate (GTN) infusion if the blood pressure will tolerate this. Ventilatory support may also be required.

6.25 The correct answer is A.

Establishment of a definitive airway and diagnosis of the cause of arrest forms part of ALS, not BLS. Importantly, BLS guidelines underwent revision in 2006.

6.26 The correct answer is C.

Although the patient's fluid balance since admission shows he is 1.5 L positive, he will still be hypovolaemic from the fluid loss prior to admission and from the fluid loss into his bowel. It is therefore appropriate to increase fluid and reassess. It is a little premature to get a CVP line, as he has not had a fluid challenge, and it is too soon to take him to theatre, as he may still respond to conservative treatment. Furosemide is not indicated in anyone with a low urine output unless they are fluid overloaded with peripheral/pulmonary oedema. Giving furosemide to improve urine output if a patient is dry can lead to acute renal failure.

6.27 The correct answer is B.

Following splenectomy, the patient is at increased risk of infection due to encapsulated organisms. *Streptococcus pneumoniae* is implicated in >50% of cases. Other organisms include *Haemophilus influenzae*, *Neisseria meningitidis* and *Escherichia coli*.

6.28 The correct answer is B.

Heparin acts by indirectly inhibiting the blood coagulation proteases thrombin and activated factor X through activation of antithrombin.

6.29 The correct answer is C.

6.30 The correct answer is A.

Vaccinations should ideally be administered two weeks pre-op for elective splenectomy. Prophylactic antibiotics are recommended for a minimum of two years post-op in adults. Amoxicillin 250 mg–500 mg once daily is the recommended prophylactic dose.

6.31 The correct answer is D.

The patient is likely to develop short-bowel syndrome. Features include diarrhoea, malnutrition and vitamin and mineral deficiencies. Notably, vitamin B12 and bile salts are reabsorbed in the terminal ileum. Hypomagnesaemia occurs when magnesium absorption is prevented as it becomes chelated with the unabsorbed fatty acids. Unabsorbed fatty acids are likely also to reduce gut transit time. Other complications include confusion, renal stones, deficiency of the fat-soluble vitamins A, D, E and K and gallstones due to biliary stasis.

6.32 The correct answer is A.

In America, donor blood is also screened for HTLV and West Nile virus.

6.33 The correct answer is E.

6.34 The correct answer is D.

Factors affecting outcome include the type, depth and extent of the injury; the age of the patient (with those at the extremes of age performing poorly); the presence of an inhalation injury; and the presence of cardiorespiratory disease. Extent of injury can be estimated using

Wallace's 'rule of nines'. The patient has 9% second-degree burns. First-degree burns are typically painful and erythematous in appearance. Third-degree (full thickness) burns are typically painless, with a waxy, leathery and charred appearance.

6.35 The correct answer is D.

Other factors associated with increased risk include a history of congestive cardiac failure (CCF), ischaemic heart disease (IHD), previous coronary artery bypass grafting (CABG), peripheral vascular disease (PVD), chronic obstructive pulmonary disease (COPD), pulmonary and arterial hypertension and neurological disease.

Transplant Surgery

QUESTIONS

7.1 A kidney transplant from a non-related cadaver is known as a:
a Autograft
b Allograft
c Isograft
d Xenograft
e Heterograft

7.2 When an organ is transplanted, the main cell type that recognises the graft as foreign and initiates rejection is:
a T lymphocyte
b B lymphocyte
c Neutrophil
d Mast cell
e Macrophage

7.3 A kidney from a cadaveric donor is accepted for transplantation unless there is evidence in the donor of which of the following?
a Systemic bacterial infection
b Low-grade brain tumour
c HIV
d Non-melanoma skin tumour
e Left ventricular failure (LVF)

7.4 Once a kidney is retrieved for transplantation from the donor, it is immediately perfused with a solution to try to preserve the organ. This solution should be:

a Cold and mimic extracellular fluid
b Warm and mimic extracellular fluid
c Cold and mimic intracellular fluid
d Warm and mimic intracellular fluid
e Cold and mimic plasma

7.5 The most important antibodies to match in organ transplantation are:

a HLA-DR
b HLA-A
c HLA-B
d ABO
e Isohaemagglutinins

7.6 When performing a kidney transplant, if following reperfusion of the transplanted kidney it suddenly begins to discolour and then after a few minutes looks non-viable, it may be undergoing hyper-acute rejection. Hyperacute rejection is caused by:

a HLA incompatibility resulting in T-cell mediated rejection
b Thrombosis of the renal vein
c Thrombosis of the renal artery
d Poor preservation of the donor kidney
e Preformed antibodies in the recipient to the donor organ

7.7 A 50-year-old diabetic patient who underwent a cadaveric renal transplant four months ago for end-stage renal disease secondary to diabetic nephropathy is readmitted to the transplant unit feeling generally unwell. His current immunosuppression is cyclosporine, azathioprine and prednisolone. A blood test shows a creatinine level of 300. Which of the following tests is not appropriate in the immediate management?

a Renal ultrasound
b Plasma cyclosporine levels
c Renal biopsy
d Plasma CMV (cytomegalovirus) levels
e HbA1c

7.8 A 74-year-old man presents to the transplant clinic 10 years after a kidney transplant feeling generally unwell and having noticed swelling in his groins. He is still taking cyclosporine, azathioprine and prednisolone. You examine him and find him to have bilaterally palpable groin lymphadenopathy. You cannot palpate any other enlarged nodes. You suspect he may be suffering from:
 a Chronic rejection
 b Post-transplant lymphoproliferative disorder (PTLD)
 c Acute rejection
 d A systemic bacterial infection
 e CMV disease

7.9 A 56-year-old patient who had a liver transplant four years ago for liver failure secondary to primary biliary cirrhosis is admitted to the transplant unit feeling unwell and having sweats and fevers. Blood test show her liver function tests to be normal but CMV levels are very high. The next course of treatment should be:
 a Liver biopsy to exclude rejection
 b Reduce the immunosuppression and start antiviral therapy
 c Increase the immunosuppression and start antiviral therapy
 d Liver ultrasound to check for flow in the portal vein
 e MRCP to check patency of bile duct

7.10 Two days after renal transplant, the patient complains of pain around the transplant, and on examination you find there to be some tenderness. All observations are fine. You perform an urgent ultrasound, which shows that there is no flow in the renal vein. The next course of treatment should be:
 a Check the serum creatinine to assess graft function.
 b Organise a CT angiogram to further assess the vessels.
 c Start thrombolysis treatment.
 d Take the patient to theatre immediately.
 e Increase immunosuppression in case of vascular rejection.

7.11 A 45-year-old man who underwent cadaveric liver transplantation four weeks previously is readmitted with fever, skin rash and diarrhoea. His blood tests reveal a pancytopaenia. You suspect that the patient may be suffering from graft versus host disease (GVHD). What causes GVHD?

a Preformed donor antibodies against recipient antigens
b Preformed recipient antibodies against donor antigens
c Recipient T cells recognising donor antigens as foreign
d Donor T cells recognising recipient antigens as foreign
e Recipient plasma cells producing antibody against donor antigens

7.12 The calcineurin inhibitors, cyclosporine and tacrolimus, are the mainstay of immunosuppressive protocols in organ transplantation. However, they are not without side effects. Which of the following is not a side effect commonly associated with these drugs?

a Nephrotoxicity
b Increased risk of cancer
c Increased risk of infections
d Neurotoxicity
e Lung fibrosis

7.13 A kidney donor graft is commonly implanted into a recipient by:

a Removing the recipient kidney and directly placing the donor kidney in its place
b Putting the donor kidney in the pelvis in an intraperitoneal position with vascular anastomosis to the IVC and aorta
c Putting the donor kidney in the pelvis in a retroperitoneal position with vascular anastomosis to the IVC and aorta
d Putting the donor kidney in the pelvis in a retroperitoneal position with vascular anastomosis to the iliac vessels
e Putting the donor kidney in the pelvis in an intraperitoneal position with vascular anastomosis to the iliac vessels

7.14 The anastomoses involved in a cadaveric liver transplantation are usually:

a One artery, two veins, one bile duct
b Two arteries, two veins, one bile duct
c One artery, one vein, one bile duct
d Two arteries, one vein, one bile duct
e One artery, two veins, two bile ducts

7.15 A 45-year-old man has end-stage renal failure secondary to diabetic nephropathy. He has difficulty controlling his blood-sugar levels with insulin and suffers from attacks of hypoglycaemia without warning. He would best be treated by:

a Cadaveric renal transplantation alone

b Cadaveric renal transplantation and islet cell transplantation

c Dialysis and islet cell transplantation

d Simultaneous cadaveric kidney-pancreas transplantation

e Dialysis and pancreas transplantation

ANSWERS

7.1   The correct answer is B.

An autograft is the transplant from one part of the body to another (e.g. a skin graft). An allograft is a transplant between members of the same species. An isograft is a transplant between identical twins. A xenograft is a transplant between members of different species (e.g. pig to human). A heterograft is another name for a xenograft.

7.2   The correct answer is A.

The recognition of the foreign organ is initiated by the interaction between host T cells and the histocompatibility antigens on the surface of the allograft.

7.3   The correct answer is C.

Of the above contraindications, the only one that would preclude kidney donation is the donor being HIV positive. Organs from donors with bacterial infections can be transplanted and the recipient can be treated with the appropriate antibiotics. Low-grade brain tumours are not a contraindication, as the chance of metastasis outside the CNS is very low. The same is true for non-melanoma skin tumours, as their chance of transmission to the recipient is very low. LVF is not a contraindication to cadaveric kidney donation unless there is associated renal failure.

7.4   The correct answer is C.

The solution used to preserve kidneys and livers is called UW solution, and it is a solution that tries to mimic the intracellular fluid to prevent cell swelling by osmosis. It is used at 4°C to slow cellular metabolism in order to help preserve the organ.

7.5   The correct answer is D.

Until recently, mismatched ABO antibodies was an absolute contraindication for transplant. Now, although it is desirable to get as many HLA matches as possible, it is not necessary to get a complete match. Recently in kidney transplantation, transplantation between non-ABO compatible patients has been successful, but this is only done in living related donation and in extreme circumstances.

7.6 The correct answer is E.

Hyperacute rejection is caused by preformed antibodies existing in the recipient against antigens expressed in the donor organ. These can either be ABO or MHC antigens. These will trigger irreversible hyperacute rejection, which results in immediate graft failure. It can be avoided by performing a crossmatch test between donor and recipient prior to transplant.

7.7 The correct answer is E.

A raised creatinine level following a renal transplant can be caused by a number of things: renal vein thrombosis/renal artery stenosis, cyclosporine toxicity, acute rejection and CMV disease. However, it will not be a result of diabetic nephropathy after only four months. Therefore, an HbA1c is the most appropriate test.

7.8 The correct answer is B.

The immunosuppression given to prevent rejection of the grafts has the unwanted side effect of increasing risk of cancer, especially of a type of lymphoma called PTLD. This can often be treated by simply reducing the patient's immunosuppression, thus allowing the immune system to suppress the lymphoma, but it often requires more aggressive treatment.

7.9 The correct answer is B.

The raised CMV suggests CMV disease, and the normal liver function tests suggest that the graft is functioning fine, with no evidence of rejection. Therefore, the CMV disease should be treated with antivirals. In addition, reducing the immunosuppression will help treat the CMV infection; since the patient is four years post-transplant, the chance of an acute rejection episode is low.

7.10 The correct answer is D.

The patient must be taken to theatre immediately to explore the graft and to remove the thrombosis and restore flow in the renal vein, otherwise the graft will be lost.

7.11 The correct answer is D.

GVHD is caused by transplantation of donor T cells, along with the graft, into the recipient. These T cells then produce a cell-mediated attack on the recipient. It is rare and unlikely to occur in renal transplants. It is thought to occur in only 1% of liver transplants, but it can be fatal.

7.12 The correct answer is E.

The calcineurin inhibitors have many side effects, but they are not known to cause any pulmonary toxicity. Other common side effects are gingival hyperplasia with cyclosporine and diabetes with tacrolimus.

7.13 The correct answer is D.

The donor kidney is usually positioned in the pelvis in a retroperitoneal position, with the donor renal artery and vein anastomosed to the recipient common or external iliac artery and vein, with the donor ureter implanted directly into the bladder.

7.14 The correct answer is A.

The normal anastomoses in a cadaveric liver transplant are: the hepatic artery, the portal vein, the IVC and the bile duct = one artery, two veins and one bile duct.

7.15 The correct answer is D.

In diabetics with poor diabetic control who have renal failure, the most beneficial treatment is a kidney transplant and pancreas transplant at the same time. Islet cell transplantation unfortunately doesn't have long-term results as good as those for pancreas transplantation, but this may change in the future.

Ear, Nose and Throat (ENT) and Head and Neck

QUESTIONS

8.1 Tumours of the oral cavity are predominantly:
a Adenocarcinomas
b Lymphomas
c Squamous cell carcinomas
d Melanomas
e Sarcomas

8.2 Cancers of the oral cavity most commonly present with:
a Trismus
b A painless ulcer
c Weight loss
d Leucoplakia
e A painful ulcer

8.3 A 55-year-old man presents in clinic with a six-week history of a non-healing ulcer on the tip of his tongue. He is a lifelong smoker and drinks approximately 50 units of alcohol a week. On examination, in addition to the ulcer, the submental lymph nodes are palpable. The most appropriate next step is:
a Advice regarding smoking and alcohol cessation
b Prescribe antibiotics and observe for response
c Blood tests for tumour markers
d Biopsy the ulcer
e Chest X-ray

8.4 The most common organism implicated in acute bacterial tonsillitis in children is:

a Group A β-haemolytic *Streptococcus*

b *Bacteroides fragilis*

c *Haemophilus influenza*

d *Escherichia coli*

e *Staphylococcus aureus*

8.5 A five-year-old boy presents to his GP with a two-day history of otalgia, lethargy and fever. On examination, he has a temperature of 37.7°C, his hearing is intact and otoscopy reveals bulging tympanic eardrums. The most appropriate next step is:

a Topical corticosteroids

b Oral antibiotics

c Observation

d Grommet insertion

e Decongestants

8.6 A 70-year-old man is admitted to A&E with a two-hour history of epistaxis, which has been profuse and not relieved by pressure over the bridge of the nose. He has a medical history of hypertension, for which he takes atenolol 25 mg once daily, and he is otherwise healthy. On admission, his blood pressure is 100/70 mmHg and his heart rate is 60 bpm. The most appropriate next step is:

a Fluid resuscitation

b Blood tests for full blood count and clotting

c Chemical cautery

d Topical cocaine solution

e Nasal packing

8.7 A two-year-old girl is brought into A&E by her parents. She looks unwell and is tachypnoeic, cyanosed and drooling, with inspiratory stridor. The most appropriate next step is:

a Examination of the mouth and airway

b Intravenous antibiotics

c Chest X-ray

d Aspiration of the saliva

e Fast calling of the anaesthetist on-call and preparation for intubation

8.8 A 25-year-old woman is seen by her GP complaining of a five-day history of fever, lethargy, neck pain, odynophagia and trismus. On examination, she is pyrexial and has a 'hot potato' voice. The right tonsil is erythematous with exudates, enlarged and displaced inferiorly and medially; and the uvula is deviated to the left. The most appropriate next step is:
  a Oral antibiotics
  b Incision and drainage under local anaesthetic
  c Blood tests for inflammatory markers
  d Tonsillectomy
  e Neck X-ray

8.9 A 19-year-old woman presents to her GP with a one-week history of fever, fatigue and sore throat. On examination, she is pyrexial and both tonsils are erythematous with grey exudates. There is posterior cervical and inguinal lymphadenopathy, and the spleen is mildly enlarged. The most likely diagnosis is:
  a Peritonsillar abscess
  b Streptococcal pharyngitis
  c Lymphoma
  d Infectious mononucleosis
  e Candidiasis

8.10 Which of the following statements is true regarding nasal polyps?
  a If bilateral, they are more suspicious for malignancy.
  b They are often multiple in patients with cystic fibrosis.
  c Bleeding is a common presentation.
  d They are painful.
  e They arise from the sphenoid sinus.

8.11 A 40-year-old man presents in clinic with a six-week history of intermittent episodes of pain and swelling of his submandibular gland, which typically occur after eating and resolve a few hours later. On examination, the submandibular gland is enlarged and mildly tender on bimanual palpation. There is no associated lymphadenopathy. The most likely diagnosis is:
  a Sjögren's disease
  b Mumps
  c Chronic sialadenitis
  d Submandibular adenoma
  e Acute sialadenitis

8.12 An 85-year-old man is two weeks post-op laparotomy and small-bowel resection for ischaemic bowel. He is pyrexial and complains of a tender, painful swelling at the angle of the left jaw. On examination, he is dehydrated and pyrexial, and the left parotid gland is tender, swollen and erythematous. Intra-oral examination reveals poor dentition and purulent discharge from the left parotid duct. The most appropriate next step is:
a Intravenous antibiotics
b Intravenous steroids
c Anticholinergics
d Sialography
e Observation

8.13 A 50-year-old woman presents in clinic with a painless, slow-growing lump below her right ear. On examination, there is a mobile, non-tender, firm mass within the right parotid gland; there are no palpable regional lymph nodes; and flexible nasopharyngoscopy is unremarkable. The most appropriate next step is:
a Sialography
b Baseline blood tests
c Core biopsy
d Fine-needle aspiration biopsy
e PET scan

8.14 The following clinical features raise suspicion that a parotid lump is malignant, EXCEPT:
a Facial nerve palsy
b Bleeding from the Stenson's duct
c Regional lymphadenopathy
d Skin tethering
e Poorly defined lump margins

8.15 A 33-year-old man is 10 weeks post-op left parotidectomy for a pleiomorphic adenoma. He presents to his GP complaining of wetness and flushing on the side of his face, over the site of previous surgery, when he eats. Examination reveals a well-healed surgical scar. The most likely diagnosis is:
a Tumour recurrence
b Frey's syndrome
c Sialocele
d Facial nerve palsy
e Sympathetic hyperstimulation syndrome

8.16 The most common presentation of laryngeal cancer is with:
  a Dysphagia
  b Odynophagia
  c Hoarse voice
  d Cervical lymphadenopathy
  e Haemoptysis

8.17 A 65-year-old man presents with a three-week history of hoarse voice and weight loss. He is a heavy smoker but is otherwise fit. Examination reveals cervical lymphadenopathy. The most appropriate next step is:
  a Chest X-ray
  b Laryngoscopy and biopsy
  c Ultrasound scan of the neck
  d Radiotherapy
  e Tracheostomy

8.18 A 75-year-old man presents to his GP complaining of dysphagia; occasionally this is associated with a lump in his neck. In addition, he has halitosis and experiences regurgitation of his food, sometimes hours after a meal, and this typically occurs at night. The most appropriate next investigation is:
  a Oesophageal manometry
  b Chest X-ray
  c Oesophagoscopy
  d Ultrasound scan of the neck
  e Barium meal

8.19 Which of the following statements is true regarding thyroglossal cysts?
  a They often do not occur in the midline.
  b They move downwards with tongue protrusion.
  c They are associated with an increased incidence of ectopic thyroid tissue.
  d They move downwards with swallowing.
  e They are embryological remnants of the vitellointestinal duct.

8.20 A 20-year-old man presents with a painless swelling in the anterior triangle of his neck. Examination reveals a fluctuant, non-tender, transilluminable swelling at the junction between the upper and middle third of the sternocleidomastoid. Ultrasound-guided aspiration yields a turbid fluid that contains cholesterol crystals. The most likely diagnosis is:
a Branchial cyst
b Thyroglossal cyst
c Cystic hygroma
d Sebaceous cyst
e Lipoma

8.21 A 35-year-old man presents to A&E with sudden-onset weakness over the right side of his face, and he complains that he cannot close his eyes. On examination, there is weakness of the muscles of facial expression on the right and loss of taste on the anterior two-thirds of the tongue on the right. No rash is seen. The most likely diagnosis is:
a Bell's palsy
b Ramsay Hunt syndrome
c Sarcoidosis
d Stroke
e Lyme disease

8.22 A 52-year-old woman presents with left sensorineural hearing loss, tinnitus and a left facial nerve palsy. She has no significant medical history. The most useful investigation would be:
a Audiometry
b Electrocochleography
c Ultrasound scan of the auditory canal
d X-ray of the skull
e MRI scan of the head

8.23 A 35-year-old man is assaulted. On arrival at A&E, he is confused, tachypnoeic and cyanosed, with oxygen saturations of 85% on high-flow oxygen given through a face mask. He has extensive maxillofacial injuries. The most appropriate next step is:
a Chest X-ray
b Needle cricothyroidotomy
c Insertion of a laryngeal mask airway
d Arterial blood gas sampling
e Insertion of a nasopharyngeal tube

8.24 Which of the following statements is true regarding nasopharyngeal carcinoma?
- a It is an adenocarcinoma.
- b It is associated with infection with cytomegalovirus (CMV).
- c It is more common in the Western world.
- d Presentation is often early, with anosmia.
- e Tumours are typically radiosensitive.

8.25 A 50-year-old woman presents to her GP complaining of pulsatile tinnitus and conductive hearing loss. Otoscopy reveals a 'cherry-red' mass behind the tympanic membrane, and a bruit is auscultated over the temporal bone. The most likely diagnosis is:
- a Haemangioma
- b Glomus tumour of the middle ear
- c Acoustic neuroma
- d Arteriovenous malformation
- e Ménière's disease

ANSWERS

8.1   The correct answer is C.

More than 90% of oral cancers are squamous cell carcinomas. Adenocarcinomas are the second most common.

8.2   The correct answer is B.

Oral cancers most commonly occur in the floor of the mouth or the lateral aspect of the tongue. Symptoms include ulceration (often painless; pain suggests perineural invasion), leucoplakia and erythroplakia (which are called premalignant lesions and are seen in approximately 20–30% of cases), bleeding, pain, difficulty with speech and swallowing, halitosis and cervical lymphadenopathy.

8.3   The correct answer is D.

This patient has cancer of the tongue until it is proven otherwise. Cancers of the oral cavity are more common in men and in people over the age of 50 years. The two greatest risk factors are tobacco (smoking as well as chewing, e.g. betel nuts) and alcohol. Any ulcer that has been present for more than one month requires biopsy. Further workup includes thorough examination of dentition and the head and neck; fine-needle aspiration biopsy of lymph nodes; X-ray of the jaw; staging CT or MRI scanning of the head, neck and chest; and examination under anaesthetic.

8.4   The correct answer is A.

Viral tonsillitis is more common than bacterial tonsillitis. Bacteria implicated in recurrent tonsillitis differ to those that cause acute tonsillitis. *Staphylococcus aureus*, *Haemophilus influenza* and *Bacteroides fragilis* are implicated in recurrent tonsillitis.

8.5   The correct answer is C.

The patient has acute otitis media. The majority of acute otitis medias are viral and self-limiting and can be managed with observation and analgesia alone. Acute otitis media can lead to otitis media with effusion, i.e. 'glue ear'; this can cause conductive hearing loss, which may lead to speech, behavioural and learning difficulties; and this would be an indication for surgery, e.g. grommets or adenectomy. There is no evidence to support a role for topical corticosteroids. Decongestants may provide some symptomatic relief. Oral antibiotics are indicated in bacterial acute otitis media.

8.6   The correct answer is A.

The patient is hypotensive and on β-blockers, which is likely to 'mask' any tachycardia. He should be fluid resuscitated. In addition, bloods should be sent for full blood count, clotting and crossmatch. Further management may include chemical (with silver nitrate) or electrocautery, topical anaesthetics with vasoconstrictor properties (e.g. topical cocaine), packing, surgical ligation of the bleeding diathesis and angiographic embolisation. Epistaxis has a bimodal age distribution and is classified according to site as anterior or posterior. Anterior epistaxis accounts for the majority of nosebleeds, and the bleed is frequently from Little's area – an area on the lower part of the anterior septum (Kiesselbach's plexus).

8.7   The correct answer is E.

The patient has acute epiglottitis and is in respiratory distress. This is a medical emergency, and the airway should be secured. Any attempt at examination of the airway or mouth or at aspiration of saliva may precipitate a respiratory arrest and should therefore be avoided. Chest X-ray is precluded in an unstable patient.

8.8   The correct answer is B.

The patient has a peritonsillar abscess. Peritonsillar abscess (also known as quinsy) is more common between the ages of 20 and 40 years and is not commonly seen in children. Symptoms include dysphagia, neck pain, odynophagia (pain with swallowing), unilateral otalgia (earache – due to pain referred along the glossopharyngeal nerve to the tympanic plexus), fever, malaise, headache and trismus (difficulty opening the mouth – due to spasm of the pterygoid muscles because of infection). Neck X-ray may show soft-tissue swelling but is not routinely indicated. CT scanning is useful should incision and drainage fail. Intravenous antibiotics may lead to complete resolution in the early stages. Incision and drainage of the quinsy under general anaesthetic may be necessary in children. Tonsillectomy is usually reserved for recurrent quinsy.

8.9   The correct answer is D.

The patient has infectious mononucleosis (also known as glandular fever), which is caused by Epstein-Barr virus. Symptoms of fever, lethargy and sore throat and the presence of lymphadenopathy (especially posterior cervical, inguinal and axillary) and splenomegaly/hepatomegaly (less common) raise the suspicion of this as the diagnosis.

Peritonsillar abscesses do not cause bilateral erythema/swelling of the tonsils or the above pattern of lymphadenopathy or splenomegaly. Candidiasis produces white/cream exudates over the mucous membranes, occasionally discomfort and erythema only. In bacterial pharyngitis, anterior cervical lymphadenopathy is seen, not posterior cervical or inguinal lymphadenopathy or splenomegaly. A monospot (Paul Bunnell test) should be performed to confirm the diagnosis; however, it may be falsely negative if performed too early (less than seven days from the onset of symptoms). Management is supportive and includes rehydration and analgesia. Corticosteroids are useful if there is significant pharyngeal oedema. Ampicillin or amoxicillin should be avoided because of rash.

8.10 The correct answer is B.

Nasal polyps are benign swellings of the ethmoid sinus mucosa, and they occur due to chronic inflammation. They are painless and mobile and are associated with aspirin hypersensitivity and asthma. This classic triad of polpys, aspirin hypersensitivity and asthma is frequently observed. Malignancy should be excluded in all polyps in an adult that are unilateral or associated with bleeding. In children, multiple nasal polyps are seen in patients with cystic fibrosis.

8.11 The correct answer is C.

The patient has chronic sialadenitis. Chronic sialadenitis most commonly occurs because of obstruction of the submandibular duct due to stone formation. Approximately 80% of all salivary stones affect the submandibular gland, and this is due to the increased viscosity of secretions; the majority (approximately 70%) of submandibular stones are radio-opaque and can be visualised on plain X-rays, unlike the majority of parotid duct stones. Management is surgical laying-open of the submandibular duct or excision of the duct and gland. Sjögren's disease is an autoimmune condition in which there is destruction of the lacrimal and salivary glands; this leads to xerostomia (dry mouth) and keratoconjunctivitis sicca (dry eyes). Submandibular tumours typically present as slow-growing, painless swellings within the submandibular triangle. Acute sialadenitis is commonly caused by bacteria and results in pain, erythema, tenderness and swelling of the gland; purulent discharge is usually expressed from the submandibular duct.

8.12 The correct answer is A.

The patient has bacterial parotitis, which is most commonly caused by *Staphylococcus aureus* or *Staphylococcus viridians*. Although not common, it typically affects elderly, dehydrated patients who are post-op major surgery. It is thought to be due to decreased salivary flow. Anticholinergics should be avoided, as they inhibit salivary secretion. Intravenous steroids play no role in management, the mainstay of which is hydration, good oral hygiene, intravenous antibiotics and surgical incision and drainage in selected cases where conservative treatment fails. Sialography should be avoided in acute infection.

8.13 The correct answer is D.

The patient has a parotid tumour. Eighty to ninety per cent of parotid tumours are benign, and the majority of these are pleomorphic adenomas. The first-line imaging modality of choice is CT/MRI of the head and neck. Plain X-ray may identify stones; however, it is not particularly useful in this case. Sialography is rarely used. Blood tests have no role in the assessment of parotid tumours. PET scanning may be used for assessing distant metastases. Core biopsy should be avoided because of the risk of damaging the facial nerve. Open surgical biopsy is contraindicated because of the risk of local recurrence.

8.14 The correct answer is E.

Features of malignancy in parotid lesions include rapid growth, pain (due to perineural invasion), skin ulceration, a hard lump, trismus (due to extension into the muscles of mastication), earache (due to spread into the auditory canal) and bleeding from the Stenson's duct (not common).

8.15 The correct answer is B.

Frey's syndrome, or gustatory sweating, is a well-recognised complication following parotidectomy. It is thought to be due to the aberrant regeneration of parasympathetic cholinergic nerve fibres, which results in stimulation of sweat glands in the overlying skin, with autonomic stimulation of salivation by the smell/taste of food.

8.16 The correct answer is C.

The most common site for laryngeal tumours is the glottis; these present early with hoarse voice, unlike subglottic or supraglottic lesions, which present late, often with dysphagia, odynophagia, haemoptysis, otalgia and lymphadenopathy. Anyone with a hoarse voice of more than two weeks' duration requires investigation.

8.17 The correct answer is B.

The patient has advanced laryngeal cancer. Most (>90%) of laryngeal tumours are malignant, and the majority are squamous cell carcinomas; spread is lymphatic. Localised disease may be successfully treated by radiotherapy or excision. Advanced disease may require a combination of radiotherapy, surgical excision and chemotherapy, and it has a poor prognosis. Direct laryngoscopy and biopsy should be performed in all patients with symptoms of hoarse voice of more than two weeks' duration. CT/MRI is performed to stage disease. Tracheostomy may be required perioperatively or if there is airway compromise.

8.18 The correct answer is E.

The patient has a pharyngeal pouch – a pulsion diverticulum through Killian's dehiscence (an area of weakness between the cricopharyngeus and the thyropharyngeus). This affects men more often than it affects women and is more common in those >60 years old. Barium meal is the investigation of choice. Chest X-ray may be useful to exclude aspiration pneumonitis if it is suspected. Oesophagoscopy is avoided due to the risk of perforation of the pouch.

8.19 The correct answer is C.

Thyroglossal cysts represent a persistence of the thyroglossal duct. Thyroglossal cysts nearly always occur in the midline; they move upwards with tongue protrusion and swallowing due to their attachment to the hyoid bone. They are usually asymptomatic but may present with a lump, pain, dysphagia or a sinus.

8.20 The correct answer is A.

Branchial cysts arise due to incomplete involution of the second branchial cleft. They are congenital and typically present as a painless lump in childhood or adulthood, but they may become infected, causing pain, tenderness and erythema. Branchial cysts are lined with squamous epithelium and contain cholesterol crystals. Treatment is with surgical excision. Thyroglossal cysts typically occur in the midline. Cystic hygromas usually present in the neonate or in infancy. Sebaceous cysts do not typically transilluminate, and they are not fluctuant; they have a central punctum and contain sebum, not cholesterol crystals.

8.21 The correct answer is A.

The patient has Bell's palsy, an isolated seventh nerve palsy. The aetiology is unknown; however, viral infections are thought to play a role. Bell's palsy typically occurs between the ages of 10 and 40 years, and it presents with lower motor neurone signs. Stroke is associated with upper motor neurone signs, with sparing of the forehead. Facial nerve palsy in the presence of a rash suggests Ramsay Hunt syndrome (caused by herpes zoster virus). Bilateral Bell's palsy associated with a rash elsewhere or with general malaise is suggestive of sarcoid or Lyme disease. Treatment of Bell's palsy is with high-dose steroids if the patient presents in the first 48 hours after onset of symptoms. The majority of cases resolve spontaneously.

8.22 The correct answer is E.

The patient has symptoms suggestive of an acoustic neuroma. An acoustic neuroma (also called a vestibular schwannoma) is a benign primary slow-growing tumour of CN VIII. Peak incidence is in the fifth and sixth decade. Early symptoms include unilateral sensorineural hearing loss and tinnitus; vertigo and headache less commonly occur. Larger tumours may compress on the brainstem to produce facial nerve (CN VII) palsy; the trigeminal (CN V), glossopharyngeal and vagus nerves may also be affected. The gold-standard investigation for the diagnosis of acoustic neuroma is gadolinium-enhanced MRI. CT scanning may be used if MRI is contraindicated.

8.23 The correct answer is B.

The patient is in respiratory distress; an airway needs to be secured to improve oxygenation. Laryngeal mask airway and nasopharyngeal airway are not possible due to maxillofacial trauma. Tracheostomy is usually performed electively but may be performed emergently in experienced hands. Chest X-ray and arterial blood gas sampling will not alter immediate management.

8.24 The correct answer is E.

Nasopharyngeal carcinoma is a squamous cell carcinoma. It is associated with infection with Epstein-Barr virus and is more common in China and parts of northern Africa. Presentation is usually late, with cervical lymphadenopathy; other symptoms include otalgia, nasal obstruction, epistaxis, otitis media and cranial nerve palsies.

8.25 The correct answer is B.

The classic presentation of glomus tumour of the middle ear is given in the question. Glomus tumours are benign tumours that occur due to proliferation of glomus cells. They can be multiple (more often in children) and are more common in women. Presentation depends on their location. Pain and discoloured nodules/papules are other features. Hearing loss in middle-ear glomus tumours may be conductive or sensorineural. Note that Ménière's disease classically presents with a triad of symptoms of intermittent episodes of vertigo (often associated with nausea and vomiting), sensorineural hearing loss and tinnitus.

Lumps and Bumps

QUESTIONS

9.1 Café au lait spots may be associated with which of the following syndromes?
a Neurofibromatosis type 1
b Gaucher's disease
c Tuberous sclerosis
d Fanconi's anaemia
e All of the above

9.2 A 42-year-old woman presents to her GP with a lump on her upper arm. It has been present for a number of years but has been slowly getting bigger, and she finds it unattractive. It is not painful. On examination, there is a non-tender rubbery lesion on the lateral aspect of the arm; it is 7 cm by 5 cm in size. It is poorly circumscribed, with a bossilated surface, and it is not fixed to overlying structures. The most appropriate next step is:
a Ultrasound scan of the lump
b Fine-needle aspiration biopsy
c Close observation
d Surgical excision
e CT scan of the lump

9.3 Which of the following statements is true regarding keloid scars?
a They are more common in Caucasians.
b They extend beyond the wound margin.
c They are more common in men.
d They typically occur over flexor surfaces.
e They regress with time.

9.4 A 55-year-old woman presents to her GP with a painless, solitary lump on her scalp. On examination, there is a hemispherical, smooth, well-defined lump of 1 cm on the scalp. It is mobile and has a central punctum. The most likely diagnosis is:

a Keratoacanthoma
b Malignant melanoma
c Ganglion
d Lipoma
e Sebaceous cyst

9.5 A 25-year-old man presents with a lump in the anterior triangle of the neck. On examination, the lump is spherical, firm, well-circumscribed and rubbery. In addition, the patient has a history of weight loss and night sweats, and he reports that the lump becomes painful after drinking alcohol. The most likely diagnosis is:

a Leukaemia
b Hodgkin's lymphoma
c Non-Hodgkin's lymphoma
d Sarcoidosis
e Metastases

9.6 The following may form part of the differential diagnosis for a lump in both the anterior and the posterior triangles of the neck, EXCEPT:

a Lymph node
b Cystic hygroma
c Branchial cyst
d Lipoma
e Sebaceous cyst

9.7 A mother brings her four-week-old child to A&E, as she has noticed a sizeable lump in the child's neck. On examination, the child is not distressed and there is an orange-sized, soft, partially compressible and transilluminable lump occupying the anterior and lateral part of the neck. The most likely diagnosis is:

a Cystic hygroma
b Lipoma
c Thyroglossal cyst
d Congenital dermoid cyst
e Pyogenic granuloma

9.8 A 28-year-old obese woman presents to her GP with a painful, tender lump in her left axilla. On examination, the lesion is erythematous, tender, nodular, thickened and indurated. There are multiple sinuses present, and pus is seen to be discharging from one. She had a similar episode last year, which healed on its own. The most likely diagnosis is:

a Erysipelas
b Hidradenitis suppurativa
c Lymphadenitis
d Infected sebaceous cyst
e Cystic hygroma

9.9 The following are markers of poor prognosis in malignant melanoma, EXCEPT:

a Thickness >4 mm
b Ulceration
c Lymph node size
d Presence of satellite lesions
e Elevated serum LDH

9.10 A 32-year-old Caucasian woman presents in clinic concerned about an isolated brown lesion on her leg, which has recently become itchy and begun to bleed. She does not have any family history of skin cancers. On examination, there is a brown, irregular-shaped lesion of 5 mm on the medial aspect of her leg; there is no associated regional lymphadenopathy. The most appropriate next step is:

a Observation
b Excisional biopsy
c Fine-needle aspiration biopsy
d Sentinel lymph node biopsy
e Chest X-ray

9.11 The following are risk factors for malignant melanoma, EXCEPT:

a Increasing age
b Dark skin
c Sun exposure
d Family history of melanoma
e > five dysplastic naevi

9.12 Which of the following statements is true regarding malignant melanoma?
a Lentigo maligna melanoma is more common with dark skin.
b Acral lentiginous melanoma is typically seen on the arms.
c Superficial spreading melanoma is the most common subtype.
d Nodular melanoma is classically slow-growing.
e Lentigo maligna melanoma typically ulcerates and bleeds.

9.13 A 30-year-old woman presents to her GP with a non-tender lump over her wrist joint. On examination, there is solitary, hemispherical, smooth, non-tender lump of 1 cm on the dorsum of her wrist. It moves with flexion of the wrist. Definitive treatment is with:
a Aspiration
b Steroid injection
c Pressure dressing
d Surgical excision
e Physiotherapy

9.14 The most important risk factor for basal cell carcinoma (BCC) is:
a Ultraviolet radiation
b Arsenic
c X-ray exposure
d Immunosuppression
e Xeroderma pigmentosum

9.15 An 83-year-old Caucasian man presents with a lump on his face. It has been present for a number of years, although it has slowly been getting bigger. On examination, there is a pearly-white, waxy papule with slightly rolled edges on the side of his face. It is 1 cm in diameter. There is no regional lymphadenopathy. The most likely diagnosis is:
a Squamous cell carcinoma
b Malignant melanoma
c Basal cell carcinoma
d Papilloma
e Hereditary telangiectasia

ANSWERS

9.1   The correct answer is E.

Café au lait ('coffee with milk') spots are hyperpigmented brown lesions. The presence of ≥ six café au lait spots forms part of the diagnostic criteria for neurofibromatosis type 1, an autosomal-dominant disorder, which arises due to a defect in the gene encoding neurofibromin on chromosome 17. Café au lait spots are also seen to a lesser extent in neurofibromatosis type 2, in which the genetic defect lies on chromosome 22. Importantly, café au lait spots are not exclusive to neurofibromatosis and can be seen in a number of other syndromes, e.g. Gaucher's disease (a lipid-storage disorder), tuberous sclerosis (an inherited autosomal-dominant condition characterised by a triad of mental retardation, epilepsy and facial angiofibromas) and Fanconi's anaemia (an autosomal-recessive disorder that leads to bone marrow failure), amongst others.

9.2   The correct answer is D.

The patient clinically has a lipoma. Lipomas are slow-growing benign tumours of mature fat cells; they do *not* have any malignant potential. Lipomas are common and can occur anywhere, but they typically affect the neck, back and limbs. They are usually painless; however, they can be painful when associated with Dercum's disease (which is rare). Examination reveals a subcutaneous lesion, which is soft/firm and has a bossilated surface; it typically slips between the fingers ('slips' sign). Lipomas can be left alone; however, they are usually surgically excised. Indications for surgical excision include cosmesis (as in the above case), local nerve compression and if there is concern regarding liposarcoma. A CT scan or fine-needle aspiration biopsy is only indicated if liposarcoma is suspected.

9.3   The correct answer is B.

Keloid scars are abnormal scar formations, and they occur due to excessive collagen production and/or decreased degradation. They should be differentiated from hypertrophic scars. Keloid scars typically occur on the earlobes, chin, neck, shoulder and chest, and they are more common in Afro-Caribbeans, Hispanics and women. Note that hypertrophic scars have no racial or sexual predilection and typically occur over the flexor surfaces and skin creases. Keloid scars extend beyond the wound margin (unlike hypertrophic scars, which

LUMPS AND BUMPS: ANSWERS

are confined to the wound margin). Keloid scar formation is associated with burns, surgery, tattoos, injections and bites, and they tend to grow with time, puberty and pregnancy; whereas hypertrophic scars regress with time.

9.4 The correct answer is E.

This is the classic presentation of a sebaceous cyst. Sebaceous cysts arise due to proliferation of epidermal cells within the dermis. They are common, typically solitary, firm and slow-growing, and they are found on the face, trunk, neck and scalp. The presence of a central punctum is pathonemonic. Keratoacanthomas are classically dome-shaped and firm, with a central keratin-filled crater. They typically occur in sun-exposed areas, and they often grow rapidly and spontaneously resolve. Ganglions are benign cystic swellings that arise from a joint or tendon sheath. The description of the lump is not consistent with either a lipoma or malignant melanoma.

9.5 The correct answer is B.

The patient has Hodgkin's lymphoma. Lymphoma is the second most common primary malignancy of the head and neck, and it is more common in Caucasians and men. Lymphoma is typically classified as either Hodgkin's or non-Hodgkin's. Hodgkin's lymphoma is characterised by the presence of Reed-Sternberg cells and can be further classified histologically as nodular sclerosis, mixed cellularity, lymphocyte-rich and lymphocyte-depleted. Hodgkin's lymphoma has a bimodal age distribution, with a peak incidence in young adults and a second peak in the elderly. It typically presents with cervical lymphadenopathy, unlike non-Hodgkin's lymphoma, which is typically extranodal. In Hodgkin's lymphoma, involved lymph nodes can become painful on consumption of alcohol. Constitutional 'B symptoms', e.g. weight loss, fevers and night sweats, occur in approximately a third of patients with lymphoma – this differentiates lymphoma from the other causes of cervical lymphadenopathy.

9.6 The correct answer is C.

Branchial cysts are congenital cysts that occur due to failure of obliteration of the second branchial arch. The neck may be divided anatomically into two triangles – anterior and posterior. Boundaries of the anterior triangle are the midline of the neck medially, the mandible superiorly and the anterior border of the sternocleidomastoid muscle laterally. Boundaries of the posterior triangle are the posterior border of the sternocleidomastoid muscle anteriorly, the anterior border of the trapezius muscle posteriorly and the clavicle inferiorly. Lymph nodes, cystic hygromas, lipomas and sebaceous cysts may be found within both anterior and posterior triangles. Other differential diagnoses for lumps in the anterior triangle include thyroid and salivary gland lumps, thyroglossal cysts, branchial cysts, dermoid cysts and chemodectomas. Another differential diagnosis for lumps in the posterior triangle is cervical rib.

9.7   The correct answer is A.

This is a classic presentation of a cystic hygroma. Cystic hygromas (also known as cystic lymphangiomas) are cystic lymphatic lesions that arise due to abnormal lymphatic development. They typically affect the head and neck (more commonly on the left side) and can occur within both the anterior and the posterior triangles. They typically present as a soft, painless, partially compressible and characteristically transilluminable lesion, and they often result in cosmetic disfigurement. They can compress on adjacent structures to cause stridor and feeding difficulties. The majority of cystic hygromas are evident at birth or present by the age of two years. There is no racial or sex predilection. Cystic hygromas rarely spontaneously regress; management is therefore surgical excision. Lipomas are slow-growing benign tumours that are uncommon in this age group. Thyroglossal cysts occur in the midline. Dermoid cysts occur along lines of fusion of skin dermatomes, e.g. the lateral aspect of the eyebrow. Pyogenic granulomas (also known as capillary haemangiomas) are pigmented benign vascular tumours.

9.8   The correct answer is B.

Hidradenitis suppurativa classically presents as swollen, painful, erythematous lesions; the skin may be thickened following recurrent infections, and the presence of sinus tracts is diagnostic. Hidradenitis suppurativa typically occurs in the axillae and groin, but it can occur in any part of the body that contains apocrine glands. It is thought to be caused by occlusion of the hair follicles, which subsequently leads to occlusion of the apocrine glands and causes a perifolliculitis. The incidence is greater in females, and it does not present before puberty. It is associated with perspiration, obesity, cigarette smoking and stress. Nodules will heal slowly, with or without drainage. Erysipelas is a skin infection typically caused by group A β-haemolytic streptococci; features include erythema and induration, and lesions have a well-demarcated border, which sets it apart. Sebaceous cysts are typically solitary. Lymphadenitis (inflammation and/or enlargement of a lymph node) more often occurs in children due to infection (mostly viral); a single node or a localised group of lymph nodes may be enlarged, and lumps are typically well circumscribed and rubbery. Cystic hygromas are congenital lesions that present at birth/early infancy within the head and neck, not axillae.

9.9 The correct answer is C.

The number of lymph nodes involved, not the size of lymph nodes involved, is a prognostic factor. Other markers of poor prognosis include: lymphatic/perineural or distant metastases (especially visceral metastases); male gender with tumours located on the trunk of head and neck; and increasing age.

9.10 The correct answer is B.

All lesions suspicious for melanoma should undergo full-thickness excisional biopsy, with suggested margins of 1 cm for lesions ≤1 mm and 2 cm for lesions 1–4 mm in diameter. New or changing moles, change in colour or size, irregular borders, asymmetry, bleeding, ulceration, itchiness and pain are features that require evaluation.

9.11 The correct answer is B.

Malignant melanoma is overall more common in Caucasians and with increasing age (>50 years). Although it is more common in women (who are affected at a younger age), it has an increased mortality in men. Other risk factors include: a large number of dysplastic or common naevi, a family history of melanoma, a previous history of melanoma, immunosuppression, sun-sensitive skin and a history of xeroderma pigmentosum or familial atypical mole melanoma syndrome.

9.12 The correct answer is C.

Malignant melanoma is categorised into four subtypes, according to its pattern of growth: superficial spreading melanoma, nodular melanoma, lentigo maligna melanoma, and acral lentiginous melanoma. *Superficial spreading melanoma* is more common on the trunk in men and on the legs and back in women; it commonly presents between the ages of 30 and 50 years as flat or elevated non-uniform pigmented lesions, with an irregular asymmetric border, and it usually arises from a pre-existing naevus. *Nodular melanoma* typically occurs on the legs and trunk, and it presents as a brown/black papule or dome-shaped nodule; it may ulcerate and bleed, and it is often rapidly growing. *Lentigo maligna melanoma* is typically found on the head, face or neck of fair-skinned elderly individuals. It is slow-growing and may be pigmented (dark brown/black), or hypopigmented. *Acral lentiginous melanoma* is the least common subtype; it typically occurs in dark skin and on the palms or soles or beneath the nail.

9.13 The correct answer is D.

The patient has a ganglion. Ganglions are benign cystic swellings that arise from a joint or tendon sheath. They are more common in women, and the majority occur on the dorsum of the wrist; the volar aspect is the second most common site. They may become painful or restrict movement. The aetiology is unknown; however, they are associated with trauma and joint overuse. Although aspiration and steroid injection may be used to treat ganglions, they have a high rate of recurrence.

9.14 The correct answer is A.

All of the above are associated with BCC; however, ultraviolet-radiation damage is the most important causal factor. Other causes implicated include a history of BCC and squamous cell carcinoma (SCC).

9.15 The correct answer is C.

BCC is a slow-growing tumour of the epidermis; it is often locally invasive and it rarely metastasises, and thus it carries a good prognosis. BCC typically occurs in Caucasians, affecting chronic sun-exposed areas, such as the head and neck. It is more common in men and the elderly. The presentation of BCC depends on the histological subtype. Nodular BCC is the most common subtype, and it typically presents as a pearly-white, waxy papule with an area of central depression; it tends to expand outwards and may develop a rolled edge and an area of central ulceration ('rodent ulcer'). Note that SCC presents as an ulcerated papule with raised edges and is more rapidly growing than BCC; it also occurs in chronic sun-exposed areas but is more often seen on the dorsum of the hand, scalp and lips. A papilloma (also known as a skin tag or fibroepithelial polyp) is an overgrowth of all layers of the skin, and therefore it has a central vascular core. It is common with increasing age and presents as a flesh-coloured, sessile/pedunculated, soft lesion. The presentation of melanoma is discussed in Answer 9.11.

Index

hypovolaemia   (Q) 104, *(A) 113*;
(Q) 108, *(A) 115*
hypovolaemic shock   (Q) 78, *(A) 92*;
(Q) 83, *(A) 95*; (Q) 106, *(A) 114–15*

I

IGF-1   (Q) 67, *(A) 74*
ileoanal pouch   (Q) 6, *(A) 23*
ileocaecal valve   (Q) 11, *(A) 26*
iliac fossa, pain   (Q) 13, *(A) 28*
imaging   (Q) 88, *(A) 98*
immunisations, prophylactic   (Q) 19,
(A) 34
immunosuppression   (Q) 119–20,
(A) 124; (Q) 121, *(A) 125*; (Q) 142,
(A) 147
impotence   (Q) 42, *(A) 48*; (Q) 67,
(A) 75; (Q) 68, *(A) 75*
inflammatory bowel disease (IBD)
(Q) 14, *(A) 29*
innervation   (Q) 3, *(A) 22*
INR   (Q) 38, *(A) 45*
insulin   (Q) 122, *(A) 125*
intercostobrachial nerves   (Q) 62,
(A) 70
intracellular fluid   (Q) 119 , *(A) 123*
intrascapular pain   (Q) 41 , *(A) 47*
intravenous feeding   (Q) 104, *(A) 113*
intravenous urography (IVU)   (Q) 49,
(A) 56
intubation   (Q) 107, *(A) 115*; (Q) 127,
(A) 134
intussusception   (Q) 3, *(A) 22*
ionotropes   (Q) 107, *(A) 115*
IDA (iron-deficiency anaemia), *see*
anaemia, iron-deficiency
irritable bowel syndrome   (Q) 18,
(A) 33
ischaemia
intestinal, *see* bowel, ischaemic
muscle   (Q) 92, *(A) 94*
ischaemic heart disease (IHD)
(Q) 105, *(A) 114*; (Q) 108, *(A) 115*;
(Q) 111, *(A) 117*
islet cell transplantation   (Q) 122,
(A) 125
isograft   (Q) 118, *(A) 123*
ITU   (Q) 107, *(A) 115*

IV access   (Q) 78, *(A) 92*; (Q) 83,
(A) 95
IVC   (Q) 121, *(A) 125*

J

jaundice   (Q) 4, *(A) 23*; (Q) 8, *(A) 25*;
(Q) 18, *(A) 33*; (Q) 102, *(A) 112*;
(Q) 110, *(A) 116*
JVP   (Q) 42, *(A) 48*

K

Kallmann's syndrome   (Q) 68, *(A) 75*
keloid scars   (Q) 140, *(A) 144–5*
keratoacanthomas   (Q) 141, *(A) 145*
keratoconjunctivitis sicca   (Q) 128,
(A) 135
Kernig's sign   (Q) 87, *(A) 97*
kidneys
carbuncles of   (Q) 50, *(A) 56*
polycystic   (Q) 49, *(A) 56*
transplant   (Q) 118–22, *(A) 123–5*
Kiesselbach's plexus   (Q) 127, *(A) 134*
Killian's dehiscence   (Q) 130, *(A) 137*
Klinefelter's syndrome   (Q) 64, *(A) 71*;
(Q) 68, *(A) 75*
knee pain   (Q) 78, *(A) 93*; (Q) 82–5,
(A) 94–5; (Q) 89, *(A) 98–9*
Korsakoff's syndrome   (Q) 103, *(A) 112*
Kussmaul's sign   (Q) 38, *(A) 45*

L

lamina propria   (Q) 51, *(A) 57*
laparotomy   (Q) 9, *(A) 25–6*; (Q) 13,
(A) 28; (Q) 87–8, *(A) 97–8*; (Q) 103,
(A) 113; (Q) 106, *(A) 114*; (Q) 108,
(A) 115–16; (Q) 129, *(A) 136*
large-bowel obstruction   (Q) 3, *(A) 22*;
(Q) 16, *(A) 31*
laryngectomy   (Q) 101, *(A) 112*
laryngoscopy   (Q) 130, *(A) 137*
left ventricular failure (LVF)   (Q) 118,
(A) 123
leg pain   (Q) 81, *(A) 94*
Leriche's syndrome   (Q) 42, *(A) 48*
leucoplakia   (Q) 126, *(A) 133*
ligation, surgical   (Q) 127, *(A) 134*
limb, ischaemic   (Q) 35–6, *(A) 43*;
(Q) 37, *(A) 44*; (Q) 39, *(A) 46*; (Q) 40,

neuroma, acoustic   (Q) 131, *(A) 138*
neurovascular compromise   (Q) 90,
  (A) 100
neutropoenia   (Q) 68, *(A) 75*
NHS Bowel Cancer Screening
  Programme   (Q) 16, *(A) 31–2*
nipple discharge   (Q) 60, *(A) 69*;
  (Q) 61, *(A) 70*
noradrenaline   (Q) 107, *(A) 115*
Nottingham Prognostic Index   (Q) 60,
  (A) 69
NSAIDs (non-steroidal anti-
  inflammatory drugs)   (Q) 2, *(A) 21*;
  (Q) 17, *(A) 32*; (Q) 85, *(A) 95*; (Q) 106,
  (A) 114

O
obesity   (Q) 15, *(A) 30*
odynophagia   (Q) 15, *(A) 29–30*;
  (Q) 128, *(A) 134*; (Q) 130, *(A) 136–7*
oedema
  cerebral   (Q) 104, *(A) 113*
  peripheral   (Q) 108, *(A) 115*
  pharyngeal   (Q) 128, *(A) 135*
  pulmonary   (Q) 106, *(A) 114*;
    (Q) 107–8, *(A) 115*; (Q) 109,
    (A) 116
oesophageal strictures   (Q) 15,
  (A) 29–30
oesophageal varices   (Q) 17, *(A) 32*;
  (Q) 19, *(A) 34*
oesophagitis   (Q) 17, *(A) 32*
oesophagogastroscopy (OGD)   (Q) 15,
  (A) 30
oesophagoscopy   (Q) 1, *(A) 21*;
  (Q) 130, *(A) 137*
oestrogen   (Q) 60, *(A) 69*
oliguria   (Q) 101, *(A) 112*
oliguric renal failure   (Q) 104,
  (A) 113
Ortolani's manoeuvre   (Q) 89, *(A) 99*
osteoarthritis   (Q) 2, *(A) 21*; (Q) 78,
  (A) 93
osteomyelitis   (Q) 40, *(A) 46*
osteophytes   (Q) 78, *(A) 93*
otalgia   (Q) 127, *(A) 133*; (Q) 128,
  (A) 134; (Q) 129, *(A) 136*; (Q) 130,
  (A) 137; (Q) 132, *(A) 138*

otitis media   (Q) 127, *(A) 133*; (Q) 132,
  (A) 138
otoscopy   (Q) 132, *(A) 139*
overwhelming post-splenectomy sepsis
  (OPSS)   (Q) 19, *(A) 34*

P
pancreas transplant   (Q) 122, *(A) 125*
pancreatectomy   (Q) 9, *(A) 25*
pancreatic mucosa   (Q) 11, *(A) 26*
pancreatitis   (Q) 8–9, *(A) 25*; (Q) 13,
  (A) 28
pancytopaenia   (Q) 121, *(A) 125*
panproctocolectomy   (Q) 6, *(A) 23*
papillomas   (Q) 143, *(A) 148*
paraldehyde   (Q) 105, *(A) 114*
paralytic ileus   (Q) 7, *(A) 24*
parenteral nutrition   (Q) 101, *(A) 112*
parotidectomy   (Q) 129, *(A) 136*
parotitis   (Q) 129, *(A) 136*
Paul Bunnell test   (Q) 128, *(A) 135*
pelvic pain   (Q) 53, *(A) 58*
Pemberton's sign   (Q) 66, *(A) 73*
perforation   (Q) 10, *(A) 26*
perianal pain   (Q) 6, *(A) 24*; (Q) 16,
  (A) 31
pericardiocentesis   (Q) 42, *(A) 48*;
  (Q) 80, *(A) 93*
perineal pain   (Q) 52, *(A) 57*
perineural invasion   (Q) 126, *(A) 133*
perioperative risk   (Q) 111, *(A) 117*
peripheral vascular disease (PVD)
  (Q) 36, *(A) 43*; (Q) 111, *(A) 117*
peritonitis   (Q) 17, *(A) 32*; (Q) 87,
  (A) 97; (Q) 88, *(A) 98*
peritonsillar abscess   (Q) 128,
  (A) 134–5
periumbilical pain   (Q) 2, *(A) 21*; (Q) 9,
  (A) 26
Perthes' disease   (Q) 89, *(A) 98*
PET scan   (Q) 129, *(A) 136*
Peyer's patches   (Q) 3, *(A) 22*
phaechromocytomas   (Q) 66, *(A) 73–4*
pharyngeal constrictor   (Q) 19, *(A) 34*
pharyngeal pouch   (Q) 19, *(A) 34*;
  (Q) 130, *(A) 137*
pharyngitis, bacterial   (Q) 128,
  (A) 134–5

ulcers (*continued*)
   rodent (Q) 143, *(A) 148*
   venous (Q) 37, *(A) 44*; (Q) 39, *(A) 45*
ulnar nerve palsy (Q) 84, *(A) 95*
ultrasound (Q) 1, *(A) 21*; (Q) 4, *(A) 23*; (Q) 8, *(A) 25*; (Q) 13, *(A) 28*; (Q) 15, *(A) 30*; (Q) 36, *(A) 44*; (Q) 38, *(A) 45*; (Q) 49–50, *(A) 56*; (Q) 54, *(A) 59*; (Q) 61, *(A) 70*; (Q) 63, *(A) 71*; (Q) 67, *(A) 74*; (Q) 120, *(A) 124*
umbilicus, everted (Q) 4, *(A) 22*
urethrography (Q) 54, *(A) 59*
urinalysis (Q) 11, *(A) 27*; (Q) 13, *(A) 28*; (Q) 37, *(A) 44*; (Q) 54, *(A) 59*
urinary amylase (Q) 8, *(A) 25*
urinary calculi (Q) 49, *(A) 56*
urinary frequency (Q) 52, *(A) 57*
urinary retention (Q) 77, *(A) 92*
urinary tract infection (Q) 13, *(A) 28*; (Q) 50, *(A) 56*
urine cultures (Q) 50, *(A) 56*
urine dipstick (Q) 49, *(A) 56*
uveitis (Q) 14, *(A) 29*
UW solution (Q) 119, *(A) 123*

V

vaccinations (Q) 109, *(A) 116*
valgus stress test (Q) 80, *(A) 93*
varicocoeles (Q) 53–4, *(A) 58*
varicose veins (Q) 35, *(A) 43*; (Q) 39, *(A) 45*
varus deformity (Q) 78, *(A) 93*
varus stress test (Q) 80, *(A) 93*
vascular compromise (Q) 77, *(A) 92*
vegetations (Q) 3, *(A) 22*
venous duplex (Q) 37, *(A) 44*; (Q) 39, *(A) 45–6*
venous ulceration (Q) 39, *(A) 45*
ventilatory support (Q) 107–8, *(A) 115*
ventricular fibrillation (VF) (Q) 105, *(A) 114*
vertigo (Q) 132, *(A) 139*
Vitamin B12 (Q) 110, *(A) 116*
Vitamin K (Q) 102, *(A) 112*

vitellointestinal duct (Q) 11, *(A) 26*
voice
   hoarse (Q) 14, *(A) 29*; (Q) 65, *(A) 72*; (Q) 130, *(A) 136–7*
   'hot potato' (Q) 128, *(A) 134*
Voltarol (Q) 2, *(A) 21*
vomiting (Q) 1–2, *(A) 21–2*; (Q) 4, *(A) 22*; (Q) 7, *(A) 24*; (Q) 9, *(A) 25–6*; (Q) 16, *(A) 31*; (Q) 17, *(A) 32*; (Q) 53, *(A) 58*; (Q) 54, *(A) 59*; (Q) 86–7, *(A) 96–7*; (Q) 130, *(A) 137*
von Hippel-Lindau disease (Q) 54, *(A) 58*; (Q) 66, *(A) 73–4*

W

warfarin (Q) 16, *(A) 31*; (Q) 38, *(A) 45*; (Q) 39, *(A) 46*; (Q) 86, *(A) 96*
West Nile virus (Q) 110, *(A) 116*
Whipple's procedure (Q) 18, *(A) 33*
Wilms' tumour (Q) 54, *(A) 58*
wrist extensors (Q) 76, *(A) 92*
Wuchereria bancrofti (Q) 40, *(A) 47*

X

X-rays (Q) 40, *(A) 46*; (Q) 84, *(A) 95*; (Q) 129, *(A) 136*
   abdominal (Q) 7, *(A) 24*; (Q) 13, *(A) 28*; (Q) 15, *(A) 30*; (Q) 49–50, *(A) 56*
   chest (Q) 88, *(A) 98*; (Q) 90, *(A) 100*; (Q) 106, *(A) 114*; (Q) 127, *(A) 134*; (Q) 130, *(A) 137*; (Q) 131, *(A) 138*
   hip and pelvis (Q) 89, *(A) 98–9*
   jaw (Q) 126, *(A) 133*
   neck (Q) 128, *(A) 134*
   shoulder (Q) 90, *(A) 99–100*
   spinal (Q) 67, *(A) 74*
   spinal (Q) 78–9, *(A) 93*
   wrist (Q) 90, *(A) 99*
xenograft (Q) 118, *(A) 123*
xeroderma pigmentosum (Q) 142, *(A) 147*
xerostomia (Q) 128, *(A) 135*